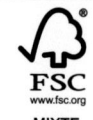

To Andrew Taylor Still, the father of osteopathy.
To Marie Guyon, who made me "feel" life for the first time and accompanied me in my first steps.
To Denis, who always knew how to find simple words to make me understand what I wanted, even for the most complicated subjects. Thanks to him I discovered the importance of the Pericardium.
To Claude, who has always helped, respected and supported me in this path in spite of all the difficulties, he was always there with his great generosity.
To Marta, my toughest teacher and for her unconditional support.
To Oriol, Marc and Nina my teachers in life, for their love and patience and for supporting a very unusual mother.
To Davor, for his drawings and support.
To Gloria, Aitor and Miren, my soul sisters and brothers.

Thank you to life, that has given me so much
It gave me a heart to mark its pace
When I see good so far away from bad
When I see the fruits of the human brain
When I see the depth of your clear eyes

Violeta Parra

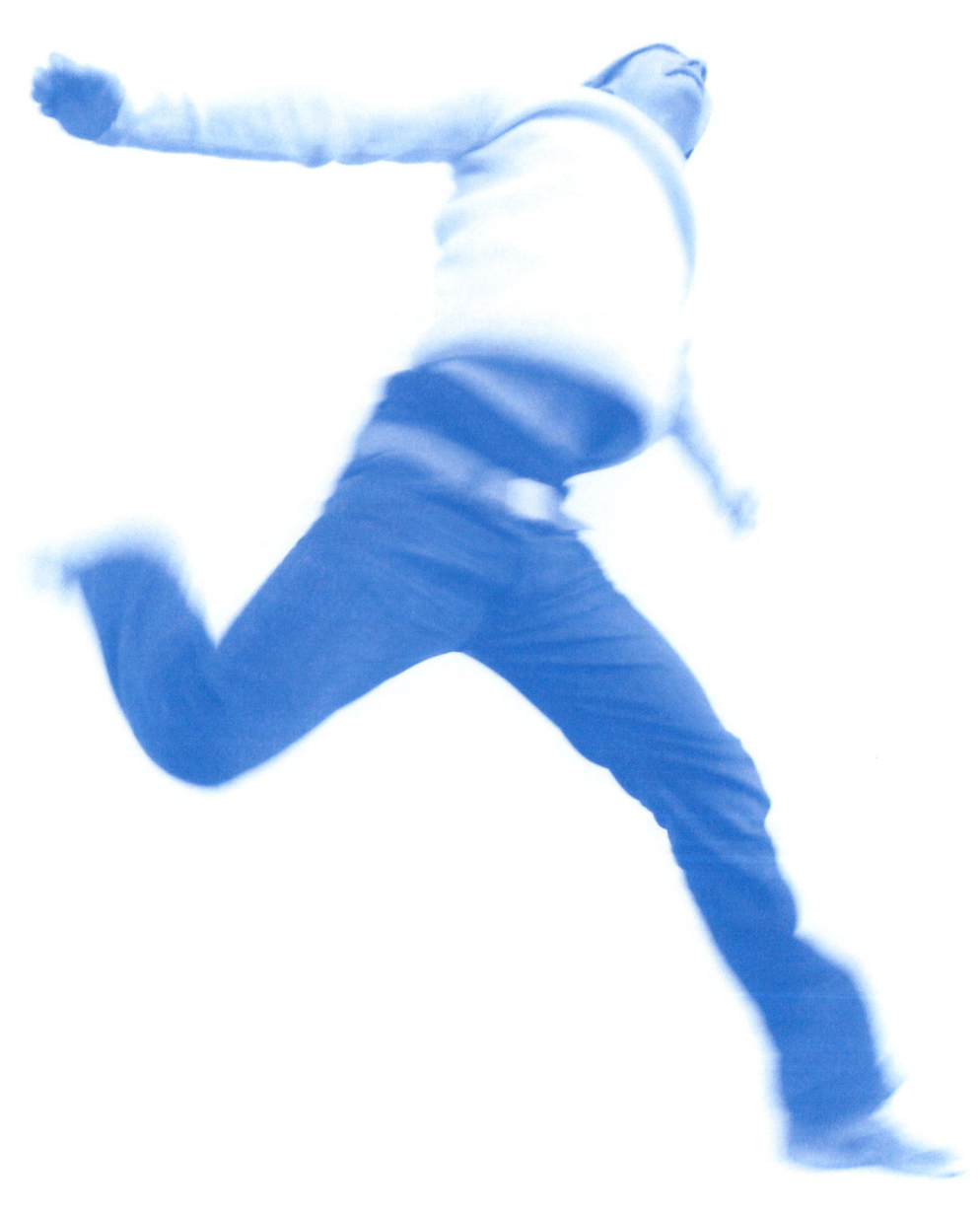

Long live the free Pericardium!
Long live life !

Montserrat Gascón

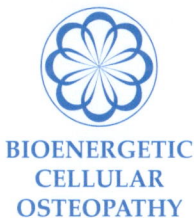

BIOENERGETIC CELLULAR OSTEOPATHY

Graphic design : Oriol Martínez Gascón

Introduction

We often talk about LIFE, the things that make up a LIFE, our own lives — but especially we talk about the lives of others.

We sometimes complain: LIFE is hard, LIFE is unfair, LIFE is sad.
Other times we say LIFE is beautiful, full of surprises and gifts.
We hold LIFE responsible for our misfortunes, for what happens to us.
It is all LIFE's fault. Finding someone or something to blame is much easier than asking ourselves the real questions:

> - What am I doing with my life?
> - What have I come to do in this life?
> - What is my mission in this life?
> - How do I manage my life?

As long as I find someone to blame, as long as I live in ignorance, I can't do anything!
But when I ask myself the real questions, when I act consciously, I have to take responsibility for my actions, and this is not always easy.
Peace and comfort come to an end and the path toward awakening into a fulfilling LIFE begins.

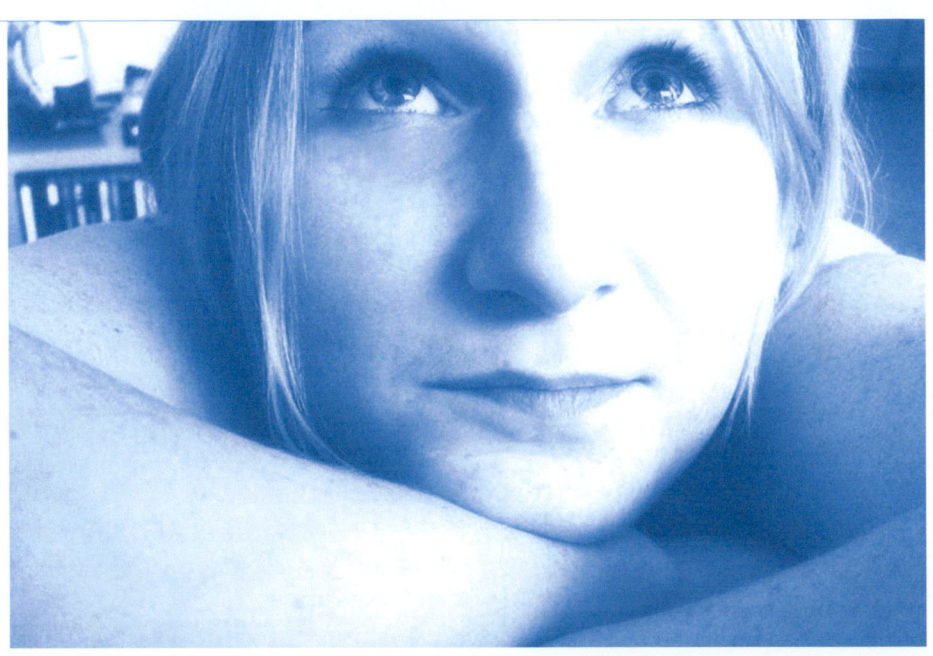

IGNORANCE GIVES ME PEACE BECAUSE IT TAKES AWAY MY RESPONSIBILITY.

In fact, we talk about LIFE, we write about it and we think about it, but it is very hard for us to feel it, or better said, to feel it anew.

I have had the great privilege to find people in the path of my LIFE who have taught me how to feel LIFE with my hands, with my senses, and with my heart. Not one day goes by without me thanking them for this precious gift that they helped me to discover or rediscover, because all of us have this possibility within our reach, even though it sometimes lies dormant.

In this book I share my experiences in a clear and simple way so that I may awaken in you the desire to dive into LIFE. Because nothing I write will have any value if you do not experience LIFE yourself.

LIFE is pure emotion, an emotion that has to be lived and to vibrate within the self in order to feel its essence.

I can describe the flavour of a mango with a thousand words, but until you have tasted one yourself, you cannot appreciate its true flavour, nor recognise it when you try another mango again. It is experience that allows you to differentiate among mangoes.

But before I start talking to you about LIFE in general, I'd like to tell you about my LIFE so that you can better understand who I am and where I come from.

My name is Montserrat. I should have been named Magdalena like my grandmother, who was also my godmother. But my father decided against it and I am glad for that. I am the oldest of ten siblings, now only eight. I was born on a Sunday in May of 1953.

I first wanted to be a teacher. I was used to taking care of children in my house and I assumed that becoming a teacher was to my advantage. I studied at the Escuela Normal de Barcelona. But when I came to realise that I wielded no authority over children in a class, I told myself that this job was not for me and I had to look for something else.

00. Introduction

I liked the idea of becoming a nurse, but what I liked most was that I had to attend a boarding school. This was a great way to get out of my house and escape the responsibilities of being the eldest child, which was a role that had started to become a burden to me. I wanted to be free and to go to Barcelona, even if that meant going to a boarding school. It was a huge step for me. I must confess that this had a great influence in the choosing of my vocation.

After graduating, I worked as a nurse in the emergency unit of Vall d'Hebron, an important hospital in Barcelona.

But very quickly I realised how limited the medicine practiced there was. It was very hard for me to endure. It was, I realised, the medicine for disease and not the medicine for the people who were ill. No one around me cared about HEALTH.

So I decided to become a doctor in order to look at things in a different way, in order to understand HEALTH. While I was in my fourth year of medical school and after a painful divorce, I left my country, my studies, my friends and my family. I took my son, who was not even 3 years old, and went far away from everything and everyone in order to live in peace.

That is how I found myself, at the age of 25, living in Africa alone with my son Oriol, with no money, with rage in my heart and peace in my soul. It was not an easy path, but it was rich in experiences. The most important one was being able to connect with my inner strength and to discover the power of my will in order to move forward during difficult times.

I discovered that my son's health was directly connected to my own emotional state. While we were still with his father and living in a constant state of fighting, arguments and even physical violence, Oriol was always sick with pneumonia, fever and recurring diarrhoea. From the time we moved out, even though the situation was difficult, he changed completely – no more diarrhoea, no more fever, and he even stopped wearing diapers to sleep!

All this confirmed what I already suspected:
EMOTIONAL STRESS IS WHAT MAKES US ILL !

In Africa I learned other forms of treatment, but I also learned about the misery that exists in all areas, especially in the hospitals where there was hardly anything to treat people with. I prayed that my son would not get sick, but when it did happen, my attitude was the determining factor in getting him well.

I could not allow myself to get sick, not for myself nor for my son, given that the medical situation in that country was such a disaster that the cure would have been worse than the illness itself. When we had fever, diarrhoea or a stomach-ache, we would stay in bed holding each other and laughing, waiting for the illness to pass. And it did.

After living in Algeria, Tunisia and Mali, LIFE took me to Venezuela where I had my second son, Marc. At three years of age he almost died "thanks to" taking a series of "obligatory" vaccines. He contracted severe laryngitis that required a 10-day hospitalisation in the intensive care unit.

I say "thanks to" the vaccines because it was because of them that I discovered homeopathy and natural medicine. It was the beginning of a new outlook on disease and above all on HEALTH. Nevertheless, the impact and repercussions of emotions on our health continued to intrigue me.

It was during those times that I read a book on morphopsychology, and I was so enthusiastic about it that I went to Paris and Nantes to study with Carleen Binet, a member of the French Morphopsychology Society, founded by Dr. Louis Corman. That was my first conscious encounter with LIFE. I discovered how this force molds and shapes the face in particular, depending on its expansion or blockage inside the body.

But my first real encounter with LIFE took place a little after my daughter Nina was born in Dijon. After a very hard and long labour, she was born with a twisted foot, so I went to see an osteopath.

As I watched Marie Guyon work with my daughter with so much love, respect and concentration, barely touching her, without manipulating her foot, I was in awe. After twenty years of experience in hospitals, it was the first time I had ever seen someone treat a patient with such tenderness.

This was my calling. I would become an osteopath!

00. Introduction

Six more years of studies! But when you love something, time does not matter. During my studies I realised that unfortunately what had amazed me with Marie was not something one could learn in schools. She taught me to FEEL LIFE, and not one day passes that I don't thank her for that gift. From then on, the day-to-day practice opened my senses and developed my intuition. My other great teachers were my children — my true teachers of LIFE.

Oriol taught me to listen to my heart, to feel my desires deeply and to stand firm with my opinions despite the difficulties and solitude. With him I developed willpower as well as non-attachment to material things. We had nothing, yet we lacked nothing because we were together; we were simply happy.

Marc taught me tenderness and compassion. Thanks to his diseases I discovered other ways to treat people. I had been a nurse in hospitals and clinics and did not know any other way than traditional medicine. His severe reaction to the vaccines allowed me to see the health system in another light and truly integrate the idea that medicine should not be worse than the disease, which is how I discovered homeopathy and natural medicine.

Nina gave me clarity because no one can fool her. It was she who brought me to osteopathy and pushed me to follow my path. She was my light. And Marta, my youngest sister, 20 years younger than me, was the toughest teacher I ever had.

Marta suffered from epileptic convulsions from the age of two. The doctors had diagnosed her with a rare, degenerative and incurable disease that had a LIFE expectancy that ended in adolescence. Marta was born long after I had left home, and I had not had daily contact with her. During that period I had been roaming through Africa, Venezuela, France and Martinique.

When I went to live in Dijon with Claude, Nina's father, and with the children, almost every summer we would spend our vacations in Barcelona and visit my family. At that time Marta was not doing well, or perhaps it was the first time I realised just how bad her health was.

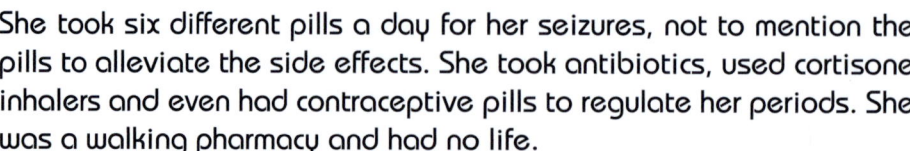

She took six different pills a day for her seizures, not to mention the pills to alleviate the side effects. She took antibiotics, used cortisone inhalers and even had contraceptive pills to regulate her periods. She was a walking pharmacy and had no life.

My intuition told me that her diagnosis was wrong and that the majority of her symptoms were due to the medication she had been taking for more than 20 years. In the beginning I had nothing to support what I felt so clearly in my heart. There was only one-way to prove it: I had to completely follow my intuition and take her to live with us in our home.

Claude accepted this with his big heart and generosity. So Marta came to live with us for almost eight years. It was not an easy decision since we had three children and one of which, Nina, was only two years old. Marta's condition, with her convulsions, was not easy to handle and she required a lot of attention. Besides my family, I had my job and the osteopathy school in Lyon.

With Claude's invaluable support, I was able to follow my convictions to the end. I tried to understand the reason for Marta's disease on all levels: energetic, emotional, family, etc. At the same time I was weaning her off the medication she had been taking for years and helping her through the withdrawal caused by decreasing the dose.

I discovered the depth of osteopathy, ayurvedic medicine and biogenealogy with Gerard Athias, and the meaning of psychomagic with Jodorowsky. I took her to great masters, doctors, osteopaths, an exorcist, healers and anyone that could help us.

I discovered Ayurvedic medicine with Professor Phillip Galois, a neurophysiologist and neuropsychiatrist who was also a professor at the Catholic University of Lille. I immediately felt an enormous respect and fondness for him. His humanity, his open spirit, his professionalism and his capacity to listen won my trust immediately, so much so that I decided to build a team with him to follow Marta's progress. This helped me a great deal, even in my own practice. In our work together and given our close bond as a team, we were able to wean Marta off all her medications.

And even though we did it very slowly, there were inevitably some periods of pain. In all, it took 5 years!

Marta's change was spectacular. She was alive and vibrant, laughing and, of course, crying as well. It was not easy to get her off all her medications and addictions, but I was certain it was possible, and she was too.
Her physical and mental health improved and her seizures became more and more sporadic. Her body, her personality and her new life had nothing to do with the old one.
Since Marta lived with me, I could follow her progress very closely and accompany her during her eight years of detox, rebirth and hope.
Marta had been diagnosed with Recklinghausen's disease and she had been condemned to die during adolescence. Removing this sentence, the result of a diagnostic error, from her memory and the family's memory was very hard.
Getting rid of all medications and bearing the withdrawal crises was extremely hard for her and for us. But with lots of love, faith, patience and good humour we finally were able to get through it. I would say to her, "Marta you'll see that when you turn 30, you will be normal". And we did it. Finally, she did not take any more medications. Absolutely none. In addition, for the last three months that she was living with us she had only one convulsion. It was incredible!

At the age of 28 Marta went to live at an adult centre for the physically and mentally challenged in Madrid. It was her first separation from the family. She was divided between feelings of becoming independent like her brothers and sisters and the fear of separation. After all, she had lived all of her life attached to the family, and a very big family at that.
She had good and bad days, but she was glad to have taken a new step and to have a social life. She was happy to be part of a group in an environment where every challenged person received the necessary assistance to develop his or her capabilities, and where everybody learned to help one another.

For me it was a marvellous victory; I had followed my convictions against the advice of many people, not only from the medical field, but from my own family as well. We could see the results, we had done it. I was proud of myself!

BUT... three months before Marta's thirtieth birthday she decided to leave, after a birthday celebration where she danced and laughed as she loved to do. That night she did not want to sleep in her own bed – Marta, who was always afraid of the dark and of sleeping alone. She chose a room at the end of the hall, closed the door and turned off the light. The nurse did not understand, but Marta seemed to be fine, she even reassured the nurse, "Don't worry, everything is OK". The next day she did not wake up. She had gone towards the light and towards peace – a peace she had won with hard work.

And what about me? She hadn't thought about me?

So many times she could have died during one of her terrible convulsions, in one of her falls or with one of the knocks she got on her head. But no, it was in this moment, when the worst had already passed; it was when we had gotten to the end of all the trials and tests that she decided to leave. What a hard blow that was for me!
Marta had given me the opportunity to understand a shocking truth. Often in my job I had wanted to save the world, to save others at all cost. But at all cost for whom? For them or for me? Just to be able to tell myself how good, how successful, how right, and how strong I was?
I finally understood that being a therapist meant to put oneself at LIFE's service and to respect it. That meant to help others in their LIFE path so they could do what they had to do, beyond our wishes and expectations.

Marta was my teacher of LIFE and DEATH. She had finished her life mission, not an easy life to live, but also not an empty one either.

From the beginning of the work with Marta, I kept a record of everything: her physical and psychological changes, the different types of convulsions according to the medication we eliminated, the changes after every treatment, etc.

I wanted to do my final project for the osteopathy school on the treatment of epileptic seizures through osteopathy, using Marta as a case study. It was also an important testimony that could give hope to so many parents that have children in the same situation. But... a single case was not considered sufficient evidence, and it was rejected.

After feeling a lot of anger, I calmed down and decided to do something easy and fast to be finished once and for all with school and exams. So, I changed the subject of my project to:

"THE EMOTIONS, THE PERICARDIUM AND THE FIRST RIB."

BUT... it was also rejected. I had to change the title because the national jury did not want to hear about emotions in relation to osteopathy!

I entered into another stage of extreme anger that, while not being good for me at that time, did have a positive effect by pushing me to new heights in my research about emotions.

In order not to contradict the jury and, therefore, forget about school and the whole system, I modified the title, which became:

"THE RELATIONSHIPS BETWEEN THE PERICARDIUM AND THE UPPER LIMB".

BUT... by investigating the PERICARDIUM I did not know what I was getting myself into! As I went ahead with my research, I discovered the importance of the Pericardium at all levels and in all the systems.

*I realised and understood that
the PERICARDIUM IS THE HEART OF OUR LIVES and of our health.*

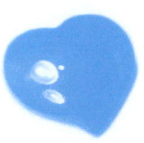

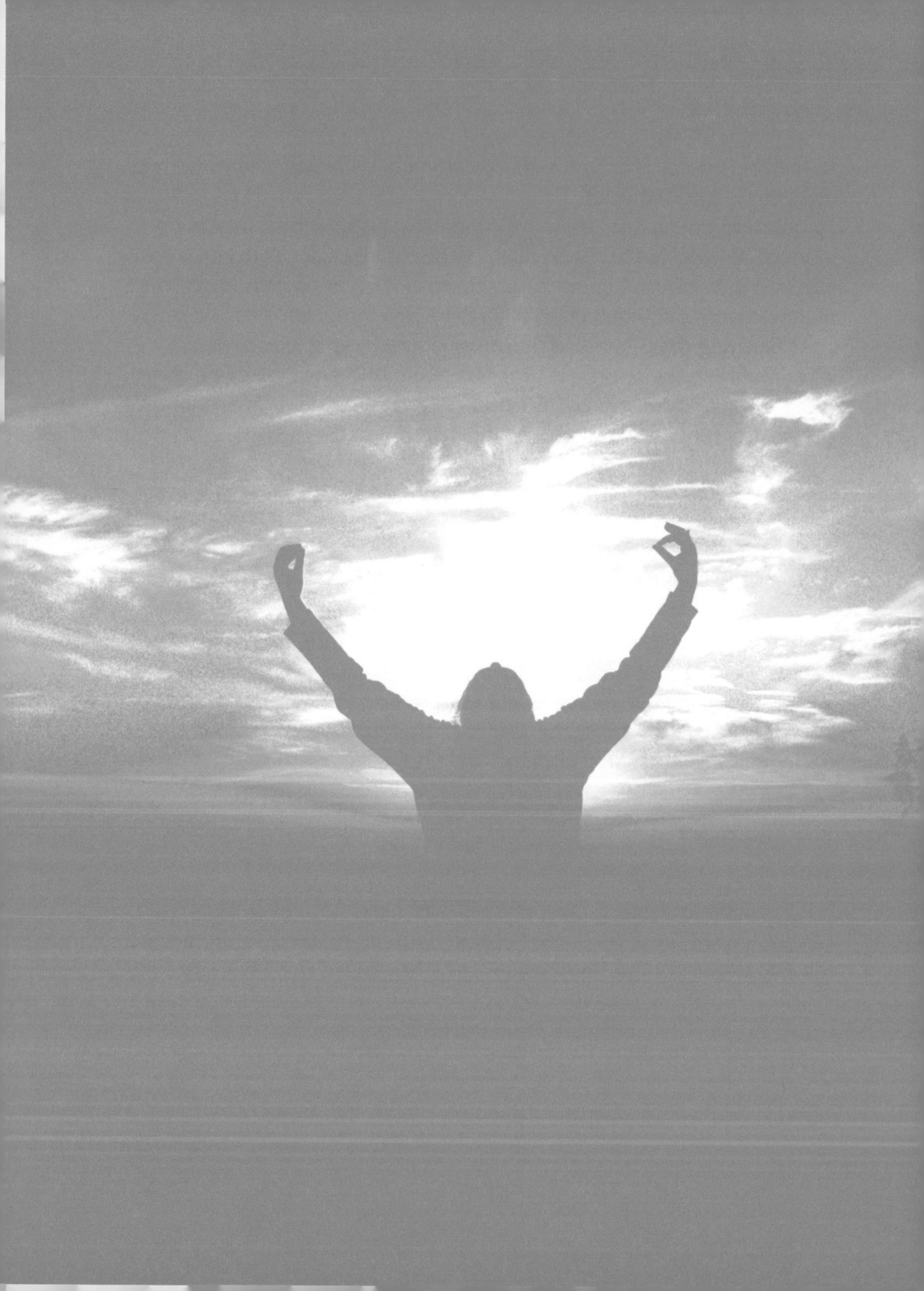

Life

Chapter 1.

1.1 What is life?

Life is something that is so simple, so beautiful, so essential and so present.

LIFE is inside us, between us and around us. If we paid a little more attention, we would feel it vibrate, move and dance inside our cells, inside our bodies.

We would be able to feel it with our hands and see it flicker and move around us.

Instead, what we have been trying

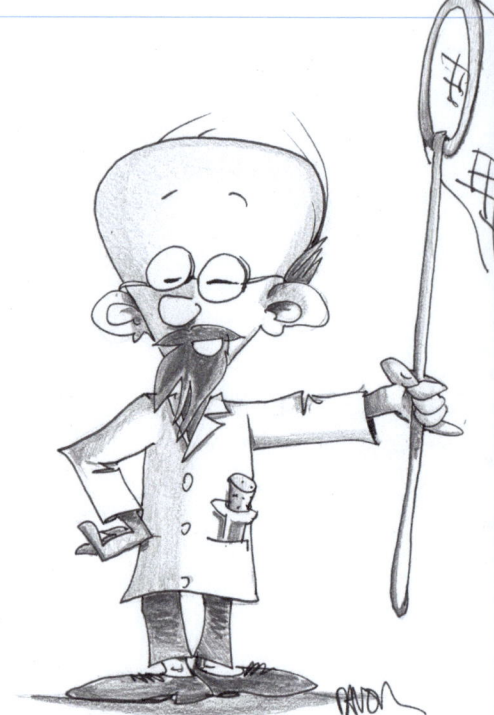

to do for centuries is to try and catch it, in vain. We have measured it, weighed it, analysed it and all those complicated things that scientists know how to do.

But that's why until now no one has been able to trap life, not even a little piece of it.

If all phenomena that cannot be measured, catalogued, labeled or reproduced in a laboratory "do not exist", the scientific conclusion would then be:

LIFE DOESN'T EXIST?!
WELL WE'VE GOT A BIT OF A PROBLEM !

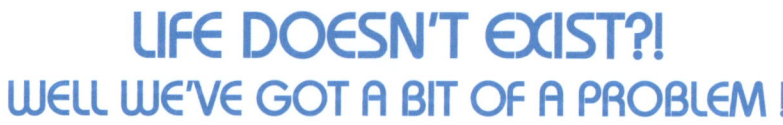

01. Life

Imagine if one day all of a sudden the fish started asking themselves questions:

WHAT IS WATER?
DOES IT REALLY EXIST ?

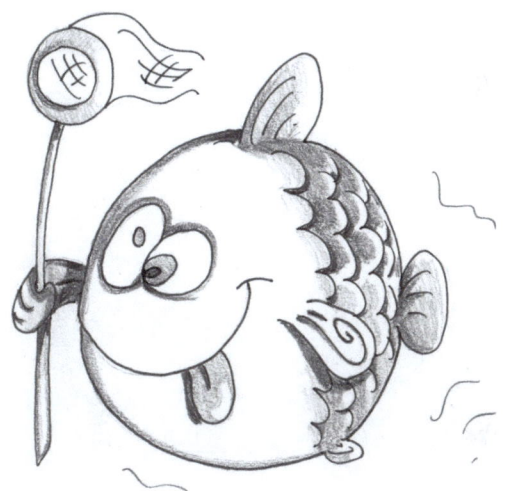

We see the consequences of LIFE:
When we are alive, there is movement.
When nothing moves, we are dead.
As usual, we delude ourselves; we confuse the cause for the effect, the symptoms for the disease, the results for the essence.

In our origin, we are beings of light, spiritual beings, coming from this Great All, this Pure Intelligence, Energy, Vibration that is so elevated it fills up infinite space, and did so even before matter existed.
One can call it LIFE, Essence, God, and we are all God, since we all come from this Divine Essence that fills every one of our cells.
The problem is that we have forgotten.
During its development, it was this very intelligence of LIFE that created thinking.

CREATION ALLOWS US TO EXPERIENCE LIFE IN ALL ITS FORMS.
Every element of creation exists for a reason.
We are all full of the same essence.
It's the expression of this essence that changes
depending on the physical body utilised.

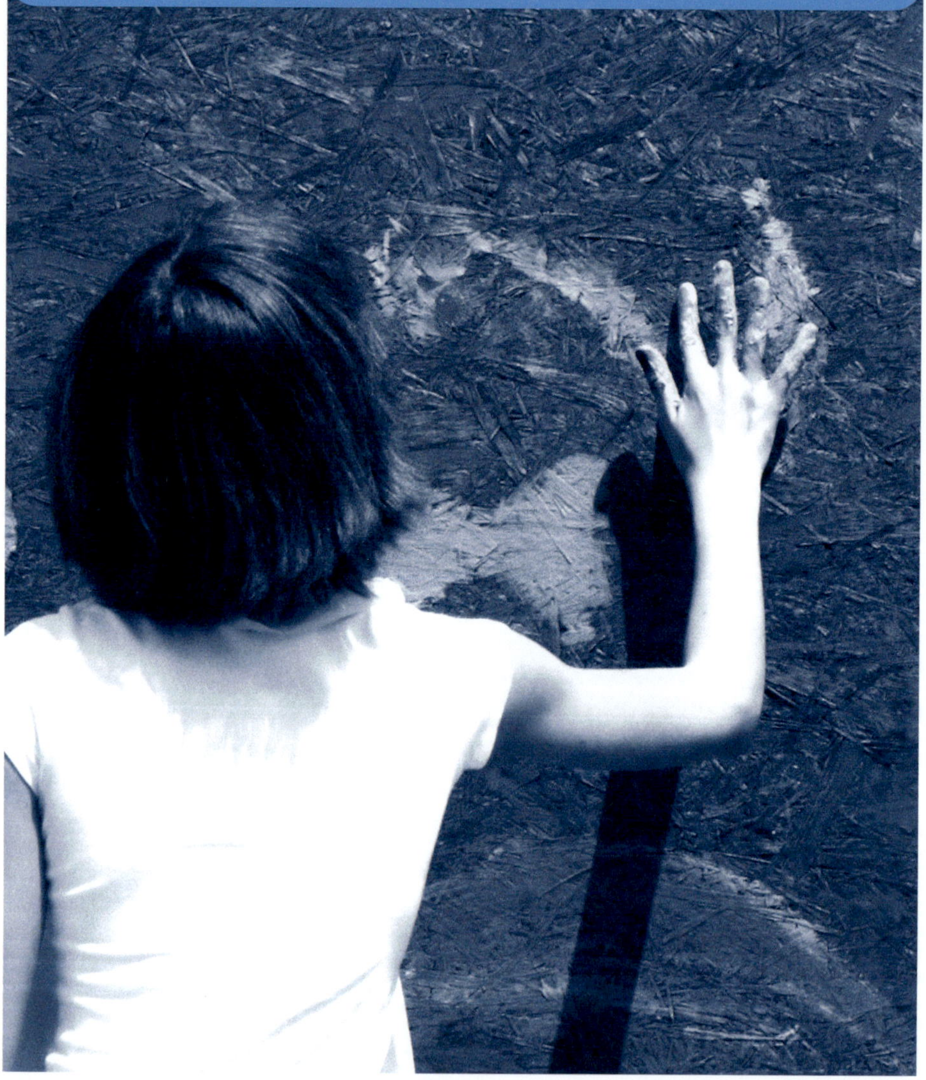

01. Life

Spirit is at the origin of Creation, so that LIFE can be experienced through other vibrations.

Thanks to the unlimited power, these infinite vibrations have given rise to the Universe with all its wonders and with all the different expressions of LIFE.

In our origin we are spiritual beings with a very high vibration. The soul is the individualisation of spirit when incarnated. Its vibration is lower. In the Spanish language the word for soul is "alma", which comes from "anima", which means to animate or give life.

Life animates the body.
Life is the soul, the "alma".
Our spirit governs our thoughts
Our soul governs our emotions, our hormonal system
And our neurohormonal system.

Life is this energy, this vibration that fills each one of our cells and animates them.

It is the Soul that allows us to create. It is inside our spirit.

The soul moulds our body and allows us to experience emotion and store its memory. It is because of our soul that we are who we are, since it is our soul that stores the emotional memory of all our history.

The soul creates, "animates", and uses the physical body to grow, experience and realise itself in the path of life.

We are spiritual beings living a physical experience.

Our physical body is nothing but the crystallisation of our body of spiritual light, filled with our soul.

The scientists have discovered that matter is surrounded by light and that matter is a form of light vibrating at a lower frequency.

This energy that vibrates, that fills up every single one of our cells and that animates them, is closely related to our soul. The strength of life creates a bond between the physical body and our soul – it is this way our soul expresses itself.

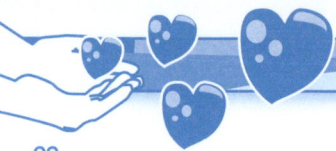

LIFE is a continuum that has no beginning or end, which nourishes every living thing and which connects every living being: the earth, plants, animals and human beings. All of us come from the same source.
For the primitive civilisations and for those that have maintained this sensibility, this truth is very obvious.
But for our civilisation, many centuries of scientific research have been necessary to get to this point. It is now that quantum physics demonstrates that there is no frontier between matter and non-matter.
These concepts are still quite complex for the majority of us to be able to understand them.

LIFE IS SACRED

The free and fluid circulation of LIFE makes:
- cells healthy
- organs healthy
- people healthy
- all living beings surrounded by life healthy

The good health of human beings affects the community where they live, the city, the country and the entire universe by extension.
We do not have the right to stop, block or disturb the free circulation of LIFE, our source of health:
- for our own good
- for the good and respect of those around us
- for the good and respect of our society
- for the good and respect of our country
- for the good and respect of the Earth and all living beings that accompany us and nourish us
- for the good and respect of the universe that gives us our home.

01. Life

When human beings become disconnected from their senses, from their unlimited possibilities of perception and are only left with their brain to function, the reality that surrounds them loses its perfume, its music, its taste, its texture, its colours and its subtle forms; it loses its deep and natural essence.

This state can be compared to a radio capable of capturing a thousand different stations, suddenly being disconnected and then able to capture no more than three, and then being convinced that only those three frequencies exist!

**Life circulates inside
Each cell
Of each living being.
But also between cells
And among all living beings.**

1.2 Water, the source of LIFE

We all know that all living Elements are nourished by water and are made up mainly of water. Humans, animals, plants and even rocks all come from the same source: water. We drink water to nourish us, to clean us, to reproduce and to bear fruit.

Once used we give it back to nature, and nature will take care of transforming it to be used again. The water that has nourished me and has formed an integral part of me will tomorrow form an integral part of a tree, while yesterday it was an integral part of a cat or a fish.

> I am earth.
> I am water.
> I am the tree, the leaf, the plant, the flower.
> I am an animal.
> If we think of the unlimited memory of water,
> We should sincerely question ourselves about
> our own limits.

I highly recommend reading the book The memory of water by Dr. Masaru Emoto. It provides marvellous graphic evidence of the influence of our thoughts and our consciousness on all that we are and on all that surrounds us.

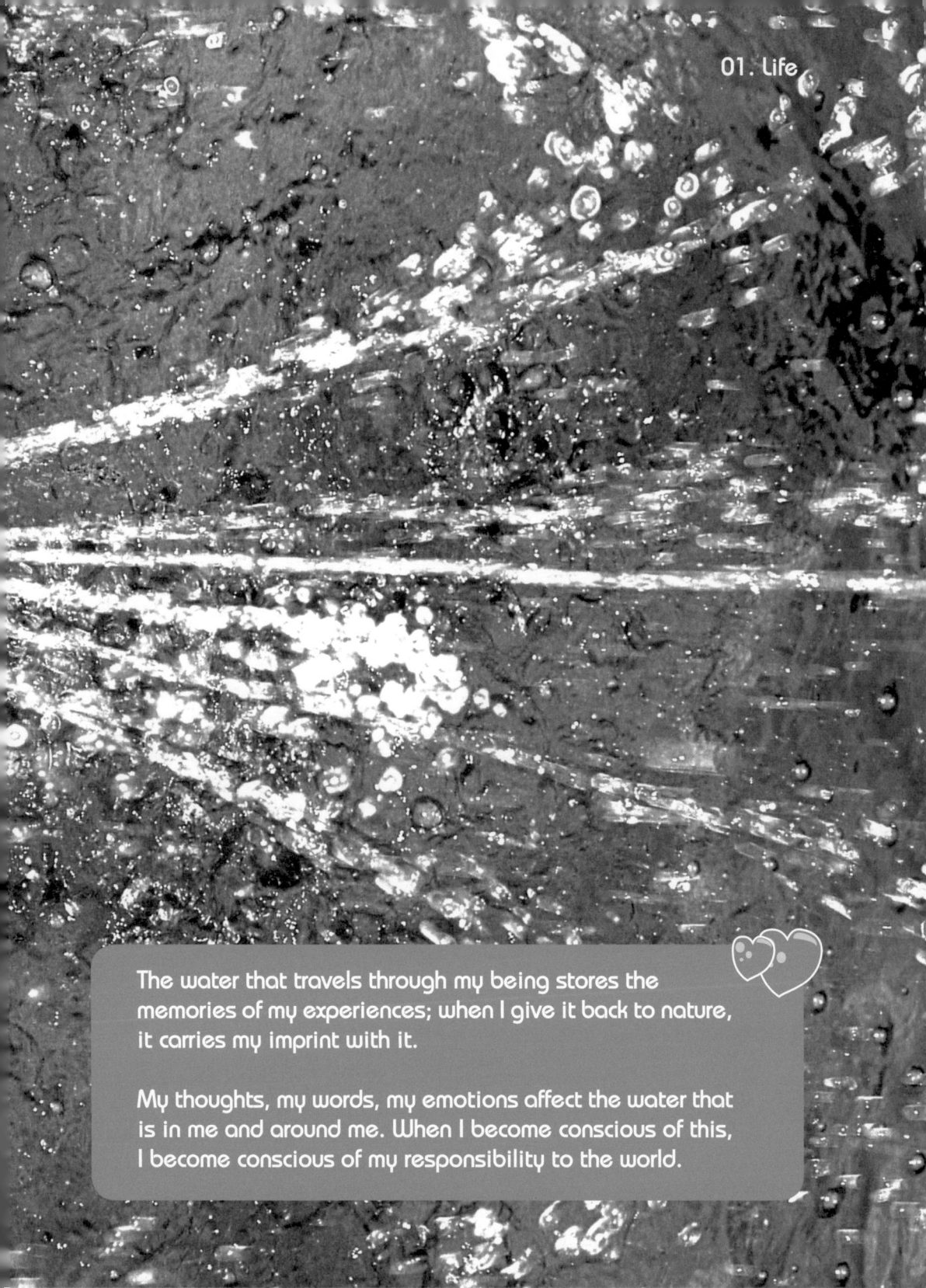

01. Life

The water that travels through my being stores the memories of my experiences; when I give it back to nature, it carries my imprint with it.

My thoughts, my words, my emotions affect the water that is in me and around me. When I become conscious of this, I become conscious of my responsibility to the world.

1.3 The movement of LIFE

LIFE is movement.

Since I am not an expert in the subject of molecular physics, I will not enter into any deep explanation about this subject. I will talk from my simple daily practice and experience.

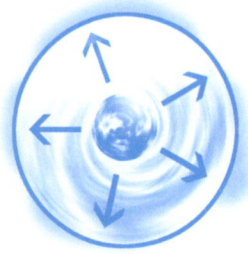

Life is movement. The difference between a cell that is alive and one that is dead is that one moves and the other does not.

The pulse of life goes from the centre to the periphery. It is a force of expansion, growth and communication towards the exterior, towards others. This force of life creates a movement that is not linear. It moves in spirals, from the centre, to all planes of space. When the force of Life is perfect, this movement forms a "lemniscate", the symbol of infinity, of infinite movement.

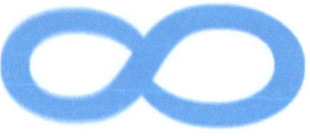

Lemniscate.

Lemniscate in geometry:
A closed plane curve consisting of two symmetrical loops meeting at a node.

LIFE does not move in only one plane, but in all planes of space.

It is the pulse of life that is the generator of this perpetual movement at the centre of all living beings from the largest to the smallest, without exception. Every atom has its own specific movement, as does every cell or organ.

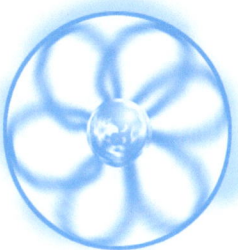

The flower of life.

If each element in our body has its own intrinsic movement, it is logical to say that our body as a whole also has its own movement.

This movement is like respiration but has nothing to do with the pulmonary respiration. It is a cellular respiration that can be observed in the laboratory. If you take live cells and observe them under the microscope, you can see them slide, enlarge and deflate slightly, move, reproduce, and so on.

The movement of LIFE has its STRUCTURE.

A DIRECTION: the pulse of LIFE always goes from the centre to the periphery.

AN AMPLITUDE: the wider the amplitude, the stronger the cell vibrates, the more interaction it has with the exterior and the better health it enjoys. The amplitude informs us about life's expansion, about the soul's expression.

A RHYTHM: the cell dilates and retracts at its own personal rhythm for each individual living being. It is a rhythm that one has to respect. It oscillates between ten and fourteen "respirations" per minute, and it is independent from pulmonary respiration.

There are other factors that influence the movement and direction of LIFE.
The Earth's gravity: our body functions electromagnetically. The Earth's force of gravity, besides allowing us to maintain ourselves upright, interacts with the positive and negative ions that are found in the interior and exterior of the cell membrane, permitting communication exchange between one medium and another.

The force of gravity allows us to stand up and not fly away.

The Heart, with its pulse and beats that are transmitted throughout the body, awakens and stimulates each cell. As the force of Life in each cell goes from the inside out, that is, from the centre to the periphery, the global movement of our body also goes from the midpoint to the periphery.

AT THE CENTRE OF OUR BODY IS OUR HEART.

We cannot see electricity, but once we have felt it, we can never forget it nor deny its existence. LIFE is like that: when we have touched it, when we have felt it, we cannot forget it or deny it.
The movement of LIFE is not something vague or imprecise; on the contrary, even though it is difficult to see, it is very structured and very tangible.

Osteopathy is based on this movement that we call the primary respiratory movement:
MOVEMENT: with its own defined direction, amplitude and rhythm.
RESPIRATORY: corresponds to cellular respiration.
PRIMARY: because it appears even before the pulmonary respiration.

THE PRIMARY RESPIRATORY MOVEMENT
In sum: is LIFE.

1.4 Can one "feel" LIFE?

Talking about LIFE is good, but FEELING it is even better!

And to do that, it is not necessary to have faith, be a part of a special circle, or have special gifts. LIFE is within everyone's reach!

One only has to have a little patience, since we have all forgotten that we can do it. Simply let go and feel without thinking, but that seems to be the most difficult thing to do.
Because of the way we are brought up, we are accustomed to utilizing the pathway of thinking and not the way of feeling, and they are often not very compatible.
For some of us, the most difficult thing is to quiet the mind in order to focus all our ATTENTION on FEELING.
But what happiness awaits us when we manage to do that!

"Thinking about what I feel" and
"feeling what is happening"
are two completely different things.

You can experience this in your daily life, while taking a walk, eating, or making love. You will notice that is much nicer when you do not make love, but when lovemaking just happens on its own; it is wonderful.

For that you just need to LET GO, to abandon yourself.
It is so easy to say;
Why not try it?

How can one "feel" LIFE?

Without a struggle, without effort, without analysing, without judging, let go...

Like a cork on water!

I cannot tell you what you are going to feel, because each person is different, but I strongly encourage you to feel everything that moves and even what apparently does not move.
When you feel comfortable with your body's movement, gently place your hands on your thighs. You can do it in the morning, or at any time of the day when you feel calm, silent. Sit down in a quiet and peaceful place. Disconnect the phone.
You can do this in the morning, or at any time of the day when you feel relaxed.
Disconnect the phone.

Take your time. You are going to learn how to let go again.
JUST LIKE WHEN YOU WERE A CHILD.

1- Sit comfortably with your feet placed firmly on the ground or the floor. Gently place the palm of your hands lightly on your thighs without tension or pressure.
2- Find a comfortable position for the pelvis, with good support for your buttocks, with your back straight, and your shoulders relaxed; keep your neck, head and arms relaxed also.
3- Once you are sitting comfortably, close your eyes and breathe deeply and calmly.

4- Let go of your thoughts; see them pass by, as if you were watching an insignificant movie.

WITHOUT ANY EFFORT, WITHOUT STRUGGLE.

5- Focus your attention on your heels and their contact with the ground.
6- Visualise roots coming out of your heels and your coccyx that go down to the centre of the Earth. With each exhalation these roots go deeper into the centre of the Earth.
7- Visualise and feel the energy at the centre of the Earth, and let this energy come up through your roots, through your heels, filling your ankles, legs, and your pelvis.
8- Feel how the energy grows in your pelvis and moves up towards your diaphragm, flooding your heart, Pericardium, chest and shoulders with energy.
9- Let the energy move through your arms, filling your hands and fingers; feel how they are filled with life, how they vibrate; feel how each cell awakens.
10- Let this energy move from your heart/Pericardium to your cervical vertebrae, and feel how the energy pushes your head toward the sky, making it feel full of light and life.
11- Let the energy move out like a beam of light through the top of your skull to the sky, to infinity.
12- Cherish these moments as you feel yourself between heaven and earth, as small as a single cell and as big as you actually are.
13- Without effort, feel LIFE pass through your body, from the earth to heaven and from heaven to earth. Enjoy it. Do nothing, only feel.

Now you are ready to feel.

1- Place your hands lightly on your thighs as if there were a soap bubble under your hands.
2- Focus your attention on your hands and let the information come to you:

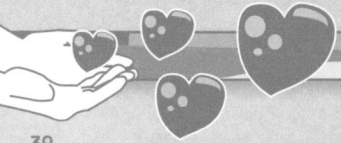

temperature, density, vibration, colours, images, emotions and movements.

3- Feel the movement that comes, without stopping it, as if your hands were a cork floating on the sea that allows itself to move without trying to resist the waves.

4- If you start thinking that "this" is your respiration, then stop breathing for a moment and just feel.

5- If you still think that "this" is a strong heartbeat, then concentrate and focus your attention on your heart and feel your heart beat and notice the difference.

6- But pay attention to when you start thinking, you are not feeling, and then everything becomes more complicated.

7- Refocus and feel again.

I cannot tell you what you are going to feel, since every person is different, but I highly recommend that you try to feel everything that moves and even the things that apparently don't move.

Once you are comfortable feeling this movement in your body, then you can try putting your hands on other people, but always with complete respect, in order to "feel" LIFE in them.

Feeling this subtle movement will soon become a passion and will make you touch trees, rocks, animals, so that you can "FEEL" and enjoy this vibration present in all living beings.

Little by little your touch will become more refined and your sensitivity will increase and it will get easier and easier. You will learn to differentiate and recognise the force of life, its amplitude and the direction it takes; you will feel where it is blocked and you will be able to perceive information that comes with it: sensations, images, colours, emotions, smells, messages, and tissue memory.

Don't be disappointed if it seems difficult at the beginning. If you practice a little each day, you will be able to fine tune your hands and enter gently into this movement, remembering the image of floating like a cork on water. There is nothing to do, just abandon yourself, let go.

Little by little you will gain confidence in your perceptions.

01. Life

The secret:
Let Go
with confidence.
There is nothing to do,

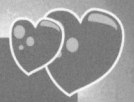

JUST FEEL !

Without struggling, without effort,
without analysing, without judging…

Like a cork floating on water!

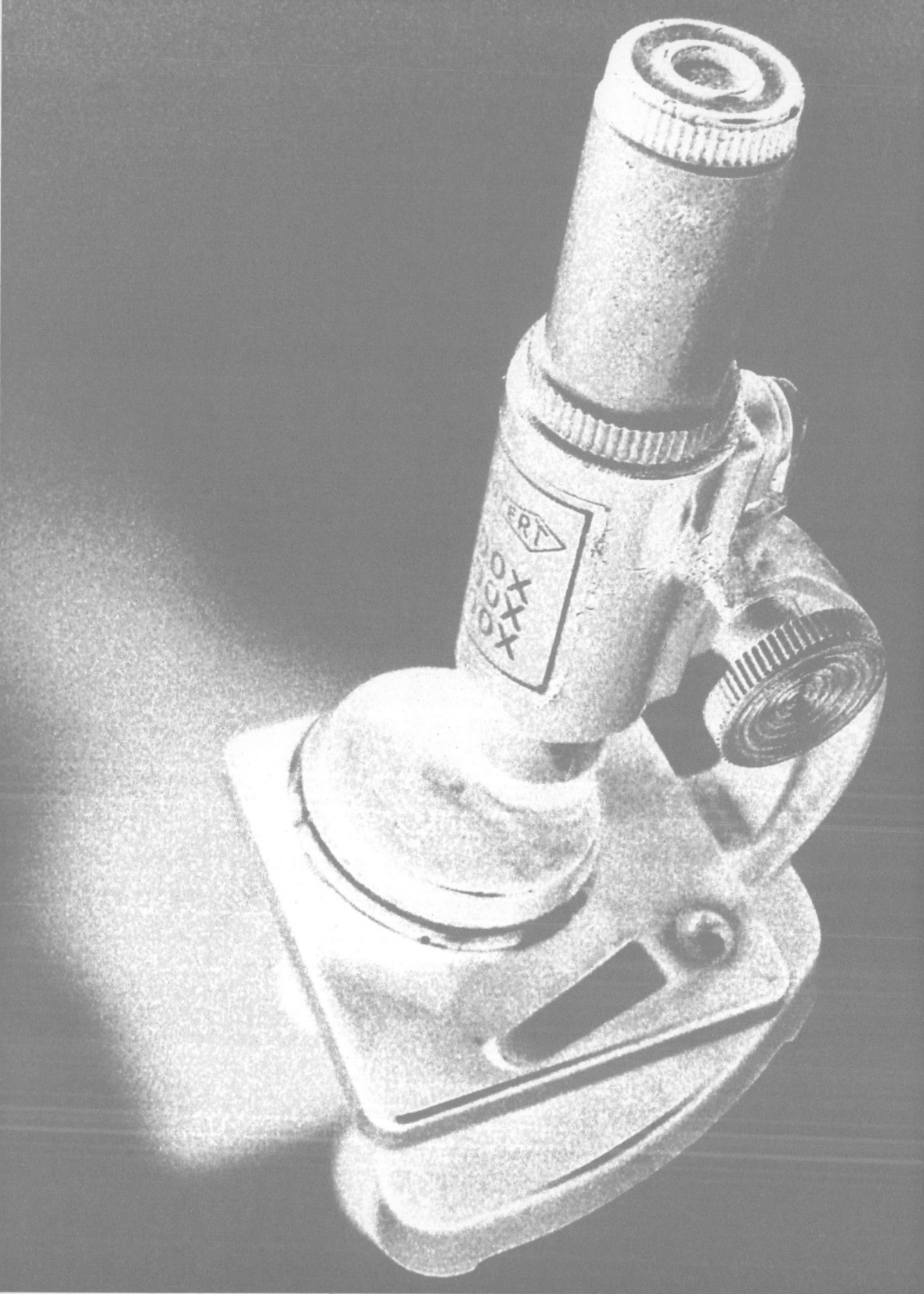

The Cell

Our basic unit.

Chapter 2.

The great Chinese wise man Lao Tse said:

"Know the units and you will know the whole."

Facing the complex diversity of the human organism and not knowing where to begin in the search to understand it, I decided to follow Lao Tse's advice by looking for the light of everything in the simplicity of the cell.

2.1 A little biology

I went back to the biology and physiology books in order to better understand how a cell works.
The definitions are more or less the same in different books.
I quote:

> **CELLULAR THEORY:**
> According to The Atlas of Physiology by Silbernalg Despopuolos, pages 2-3:
>
> - All living organisms are composed of cells and their components.
> - All cells are similar in their chemical structure.
> - New cells are formed by the cellular division of existing cells.
> - The activity of an organism is the sum of activities and interaction of its cells.
>
> **THE CELL IS THE SMALLEST UNIT OF ALL LIVING BEINGS.**
>
> The cellular membrane separates the interior of the cell from the outside. Inside the cell is where the cytoplasm is found along with cellular organelles, which are also surrounded by other membranes.

In various books I have found three universal biological laws that apply to all living beings.

The simple clarity of these three biological laws has allowed me to understand how we function.

2.2 Fundamental biological laws

Every living cell of any species is endowed with:

A/ MEMORY

Composed of:
- the genetic patrimony specific to each species.
- the cultural, social, educational, familial, and ancestral memory.
- the phylogenetic memory; that is, the memory of the entire evolution of living beings, from the first cell that created the first unicellular being, followed by the fish, the amphibians, the reptiles, the birds, the quadruped mammals, the bipeds to man.
- the ontogenetic memory; that is, of the entire evolution of Humans.

And all of this is contained inside each of our cells !

At the beginning we are the result of the union of two single-cell beings: the ovule of our mother and the sperm cell or spermatozoon of our father.

We then swim like fish in the amniotic fluid of our mother.

During the embryonic period, we are surprisingly similar to any other embryo of any other species.

From the third month on we become a foetus with human characteristics.

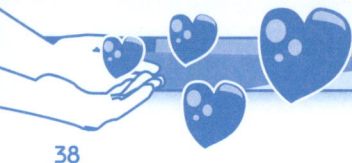

From the moment we are born until we take our first steps, we go through different stages that are a reminder of these memories: slithering, balancing, crawling, rolling, and finally standing up and walking.

All these different stages the child goes through are necessary for his or her psychomotor development because each stage creates specific neurological circuits that will allow the child to first walk, then talk, and finally think "correctly", in the physiological sense of the word.
I highly recommend reading the work of Beatriz Padovan and her Neurofunctional Reorganisation Method (www.padovan.pro.br).

B/ CONCIOUSNESS

Physiologically, the cell "knows" in each moment exactly how it should react, the metabolic changes it has to go through, the chemical reactions, the mode of communication, etc., in order to succeed in its mission to LIVE.

In case of difficulties, the cell will do anything to survive.

It is as if each cell had a small brain that allowed it to do exactly what it needs to do.
And what if this small brain were nothing more than the pure intelligence of LIFE that lives inside each cell?
This wisdom, this knowledge is inside the human being from birth.

Knowledge:
In Spanish: Conocimiento
In French: Connaissance
In Catalan: Coneixement
Con in these languages means with
Nacimiento = naissance = naixement = birth
We are born with it, with knowledge.

02. The Cell

All living cells are governed by:
C/ THE LAW OF DILATION- RETRACTION

This law deserves an entire chapter of its own.
This law is so important to me that I would say it is the basis of my work; it is the foundation of LIFE.

It is a fundamental law of biology discovered at the beginning of the twentieth century by the French doctor, Claude Sigaud, and completed by Dr. Louis Corman of Nantes (the father of morphopsychology). According to Corman:

"The expansion/dilation instinct:
The main priority of a cell (of any living being) is to communicate with its environment, to exchange in order to grow, to nourish itself from all that the exterior provides and to expand its vital space more and more, radiating its force all around itself.

The conservation/retraction instinct:
This is the process by which the cell (of any living being) breaks contact with the external environment when there is a perceived threat of danger and retracts, thus concentrating its inner force in order to use it for the essential vital functions of life in order to survive."

Corman, Louis, 1987. Visages et Caractères, pp. 20-23. Paris: Presses Universitaires de France.

In reality, the objective of all cells is to LIVE at all cost. The cell's drive to live makes it dilate, thereby increasing the area of contact with its surroundings, and in turn allowing more exchanges to take place, maximizing the use of all the elements that surround it.

When the cell environment becomes harmful and dangerous to its survival, its only way to protect itself is to retract, thus reducing to the maximum its contact surface and its exchanges with the exterior. This way the cell concentrates all its energy, its life force, inside in order to protect itself and survive.

To cite Corman:
"Retraction should not be seen in opposition to dilation, as if they were two antagonistic states. In reality, it is not a state but rather an active process, a movement towards the inside. Instead of expanding to the outside in a movement of growth of its vital space, the energy flows to the inside; it concentrates on the inside of the organism in order to attend to the vital functions and to maintain LIFE.

Given its importance, I cannot emphasise enough: retraction is not atrophy, neither is it a diminution in the vitality of the organism, but rather an active defence mechanism, correlated with hypersensitivity. As the organism perceives the slightest vibrations in the exterior environment and their minor repercussions on the internal organs, its remedy is to suspend exchanges. The organism manifests this sensitive defence mechanism at all levels. It starts first at the skin level, as this is the organ that is most directly exposed to the aggressions of the external environment, and for that reason, it is the first one to react.

It should be noted that all retracted areas have this heightened sensitivity; they are very sensitive to touch, even to a slight touch, as well as to cold and heat.
Retraction is regulated depending on the need for defence. Its purpose is to reduce exchanges with the environment when it is perceived to be potentially harmful: reduce but not suppress.
Retraction can be a temporary response to a situation of transitory danger in the areas where the organism is directly threatened, but it can also become long-lasting if the threat is permanent."

Corman, Louis, 1987. Visages et Caractères. Paris: Presses Universitaires de France.

02. The Cell

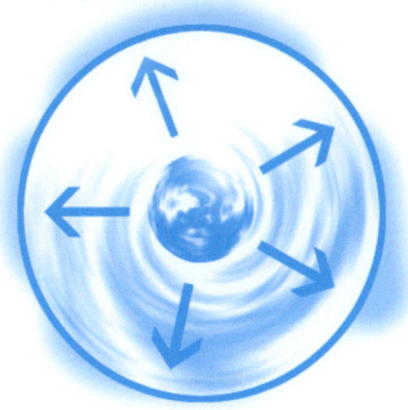

> When one lives fully, one vibrates
> But often instead of living,
> ## All we do is survive.

I open myself to grow,
I close to protect myself,
All of our cells and all of our systems work the same way.
All that opens does so towards LIFE,
All that closes does so for survival, even to the extreme of death.
Ideally this opening / closing process should always be flexible and functioning well so that it can be used when it is necessary, during a temporary dangerous situation, and for nothing more.

BUT...

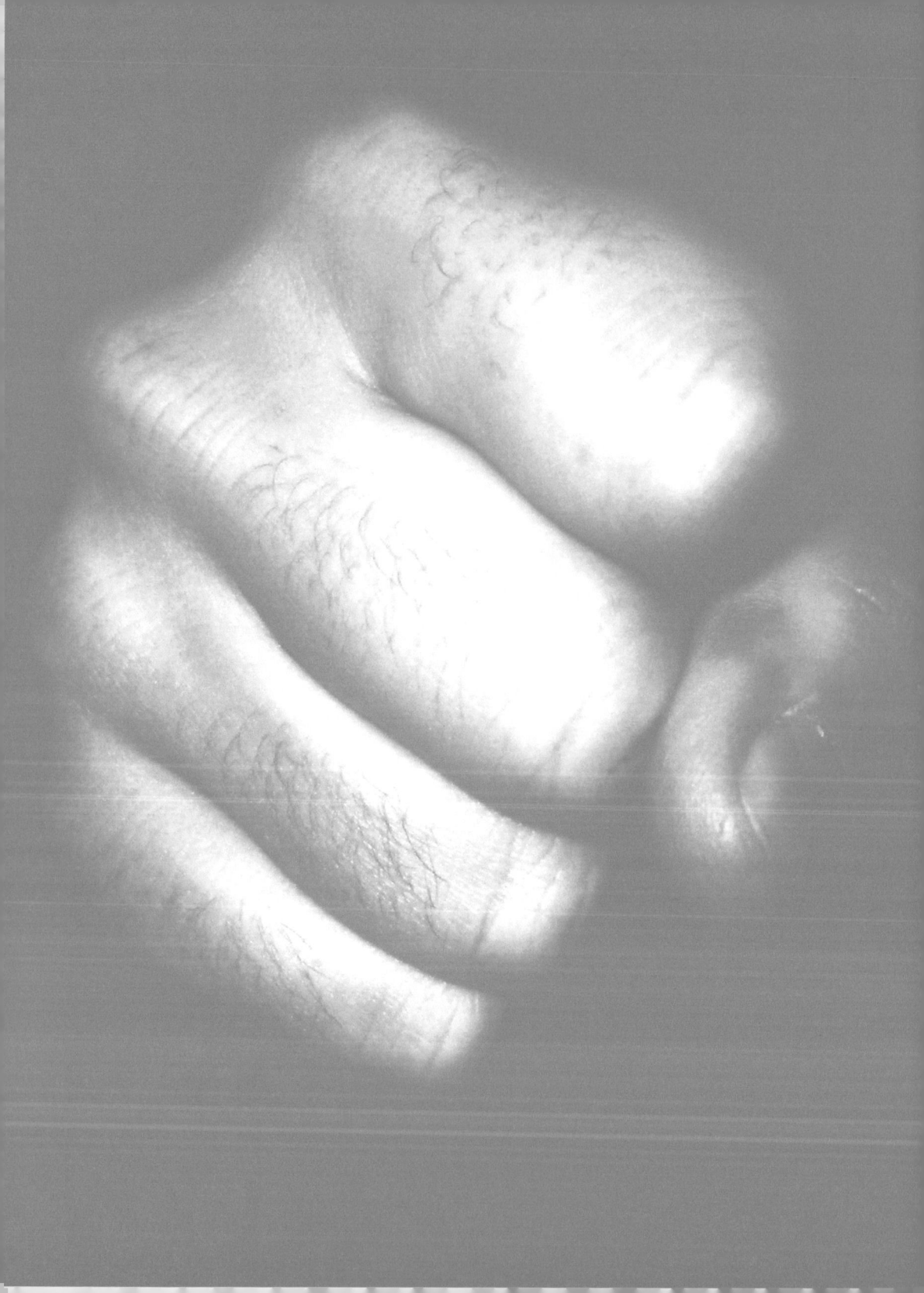

fear

Chapter 3.

Blocks Life on the inside of our cells.

HOW?

A great French philosopher said:

Fear is the worst disease, as it contains all of them.

We block LIFE when we feel threatened or in danger, when we feel scared. Our cell membranes retract and close up, not allowing the cells to do their job correctly.

LIFE stays there locked inside, waiting for better days to come when it can come out, waiting for us to become conscious or for someone to help us to release it so that it can continue its path.

Is it that simple?

Yes!
LIFE is simple.
LIFE only wants to flow freely within us, through us and among us in order for us to be fully alive and vibrate.

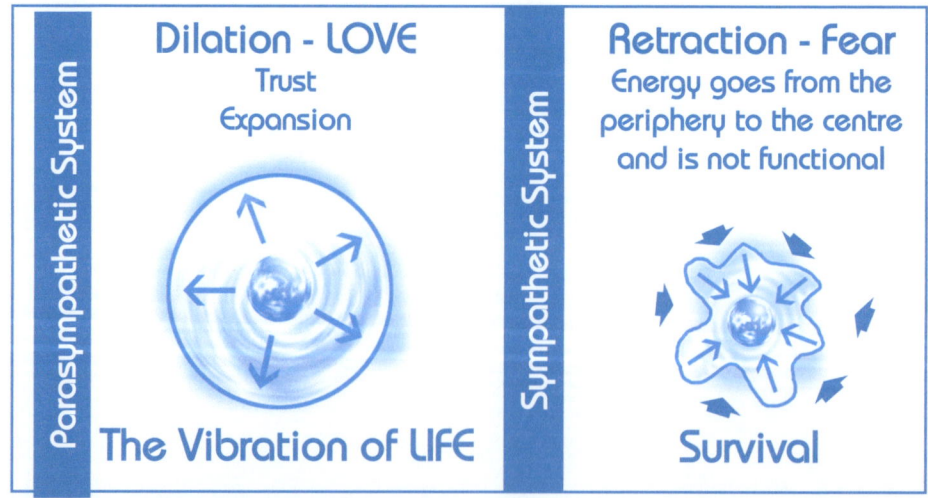

BUT...
We are all masters in the art of **COMPLICATING LIFE**.
We all complicate our lives, and as a result, we complicate the lives of those around us:
in our society, our country,
on the earth and in the entire universe.

Bravo!

We also block life because of our ignorance:
Ignorance about who we are and what life is; ignorance about life's importance and its role in our health; about how it connects all living beings; and about its essential functioning and sacred essence.

Ignorance exists also because we do not know that we block life and consequently, we do not know how to unblock it either.
We make it live a poor life ... our life!

> When we feel we are in danger
> We block LIFE inside of our cells
> And this happens because of our cell membrane.

> **LIFE:**
> It knows everything, even if we do not realise it.
> It is much more subtle and intelligent than our brain.
> It knows long before we think.
> It stores within itself the memory of EVERYTHING.
> It speaks to us with the language of Wisdom but for what, if we do not listen?

The worst kind of deafness is that of one who does not wish to hear.

Fear is the first emotion to appear when we forget who we are, when we forget our divinity.

We are divine beings, incarnated gods, and unlimited beings, whose only mission is to experience life in a physical body of flesh and bones.

We are light beings living in a material world in order to evolve and become realised souls.

Forgetting that our true essence is unlimited, fear appears and causes our physical form/body to retract and limit itself, which prevents us from freely expressing our divine essence.

Fear of death, of pain and of separation, given that I think and affirm that I am no more than this physical body that surrounds and encumbers me.
Fear of losing my loved ones, my children, my family.
Fear of illness, of microbes that I do not understand.
Fear of lacking money, of losing what I have.
Fear of not being loved, of being abandoned, of being betrayed, of not being recognised, of being judged by others, fear of exile.
Fear of desperation, of loneliness, and of solitude.

FEAR, FEAR, FEAR
HOW CAN A GOD BE AFRAID?

03. Fear

Life is pure experience, and the only mistake that we can make is to not to live this experience.
Experiences are neither good nor bad; it all depends on our perspective.

The vibration of life is happiness.

Sadness is related to fear, which is the opposite of love.

How can a God be sad or afraid?

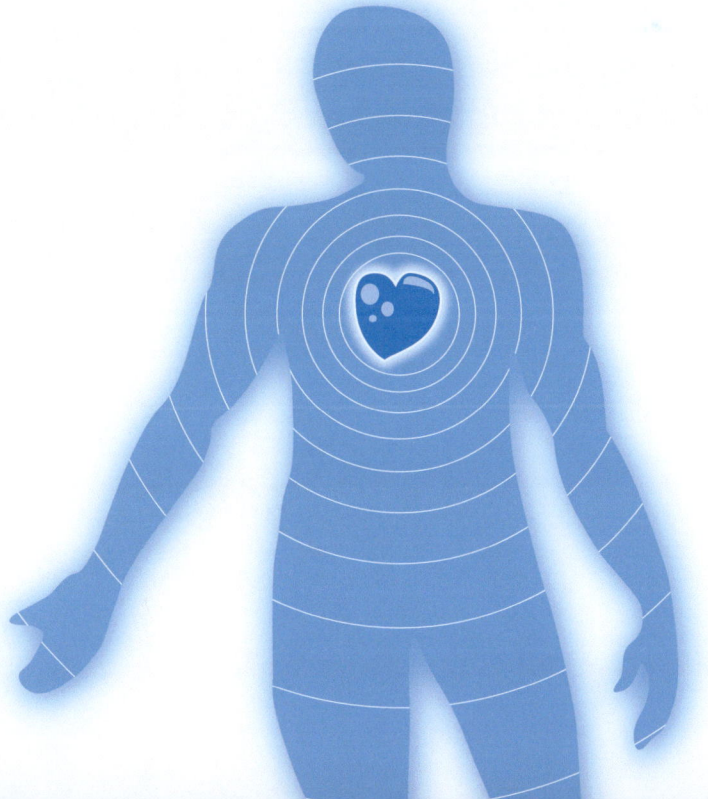

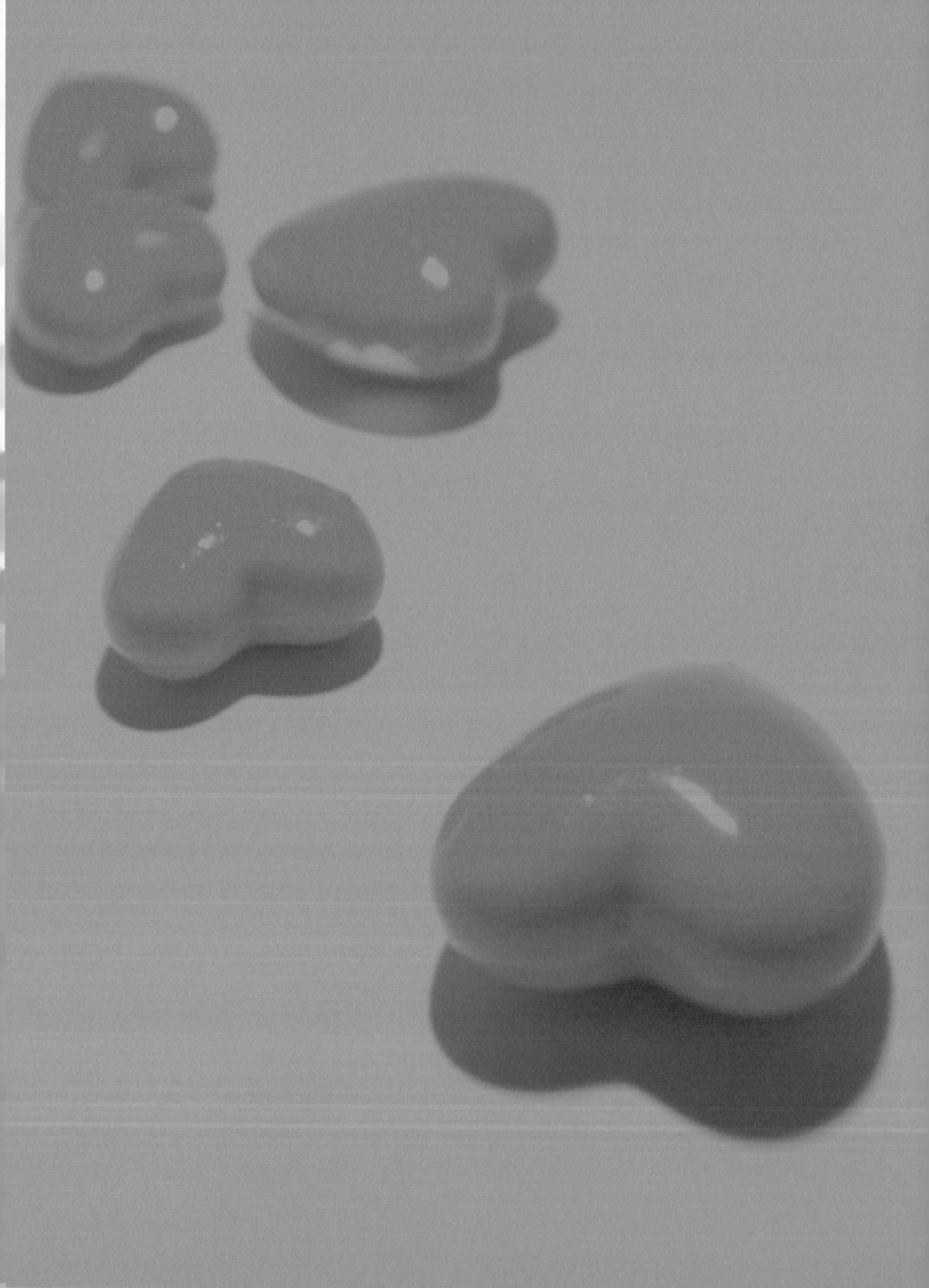

The Pericardium

Chapter 4.

4.1 Why the Pericardium?

As I explained before, when I submitted my Osteopathy thesis proposal on "Osteopathy in the treatment of epileptic seizures" I was turned down. A single case was not considered exhaustive research. So, I had to quickly change the subject, and I chose to study the Pericardium, not knowing what I was getting into.

The title of my thesis was:
"The Pericardium, emotions and
the relationship with the first rib"

Indeed, I had observed in my daily practice that many of the patients that came to see me with upper limb pathologies (tendonitis, neuralgias in the shoulder, elbow, wrist and hand) had osteopathic lesion in the Pericardium, which means there was a restriction of mobility. To be clearer, they had a constricted heart.
I did a study with 100 people, and 90% of them confessed during the interview that before their pain began they had had some type of trauma or emotional stress, something that had 'touched their heart'. It was during this study and while I was working on my thesis that I realised the importance of the Pericardium.

I found myself struck by this organ, which on the surface seemed to be insignificant, but there was a hidden meaning to be discovered.

So I invite you to discover the Pericardium or to rediscover it, but this time with different eyes, with the eyes of a child and with eyes of the heart. If you are able to do so, you will never see LIFE and HEALTH in the same way again.

How many times a day do we hear people talk about psychosomatic diseases? How many articles have we read in the press on this subject?

We are convinced that stress affects our health and that the pace of life today makes us ill. The diseases we cannot explain are classified as psychosomatic. After a stressful event or an emotional trauma, we do not feel well.

There are songs and poems that talk about love and the pain of the heart. Popular cultural expressions and ancient folk wisdom describe the different states of the heart and illustrate in a graphic way the different experiences of life and their repercussions on the Pericardium/heart:

- The heart tied in a knot
- A heart of stone
- A sinking heart
- A heart of gold
- Heartfelt

- Light-hearted
- Broken-hearted
- To feel your heart in your throat
- A happy heart
- My heart is exploding

The heart has reasons that reason ignores.

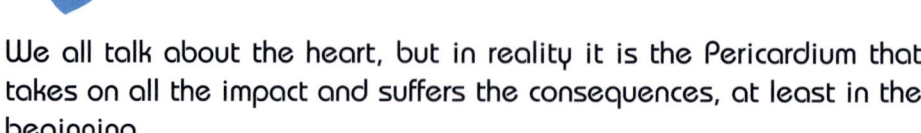

We all talk about the heart, but in reality it is the Pericardium that takes on all the impact and suffers the consequences, at least in the beginning.

It is the Pericardium that manages the stress and all the aggressions the heart receives: the big happy experiences that make our heart explode, as well as the hard blows that leave permanent scars on our heart / Pericardium / body.

The Pericardium is there precisely to prevent the heart from becoming distracted from its vital function, which would endanger our life.

I would like to draw again the link between poetry and science. Throughout my work in this area, I have seen on many occasions how poetry and science talk about the same thing, but in very different terms.

Separating them and compartmentalizing them is to lose the essence.

Humans are made of elements, from the subtlest to the densest. And it is the union and the harmony of these physical, emotional and spiritual elements that allows us to enjoy good health.

It is this magical totality that makes us who we are:
human beings

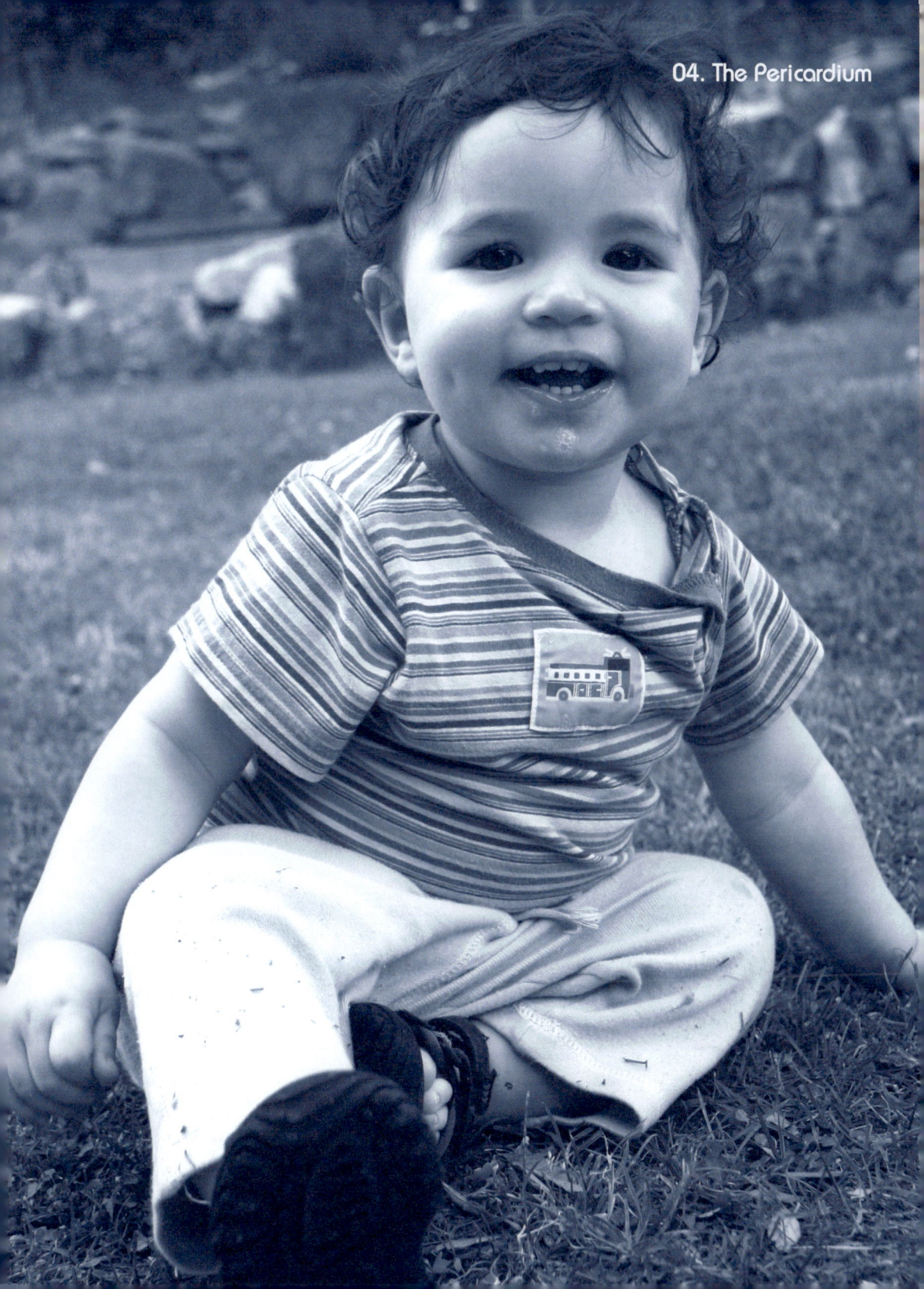

04. The Pericardium

4.2 What is the Pericardium?

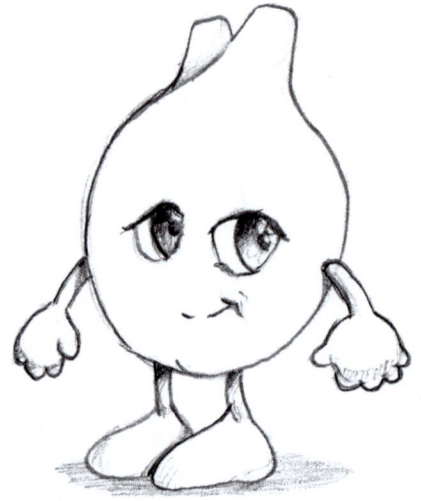

Anatomically speaking, the Pericardium is the membrane that surrounds and protects the heart.

The heart is the vital organ par excellence. In the embryo, it is the first organ that is formed and if it stops, we die.

> We can survive when our brain stops functioning, with only one lung or one kidney, but not without the heart. Can you imagine the responsibility of the Pericardium, which is the HEART's bodyguard?

Returning to the anatomical description:
"The Pericardium is the fibro serous sac, which envelopes the heart and the roots of the great blood vessels.

It is composed of two parts:
The serous Pericardium: it is located in the internal part of this sac, in direct contact with the heart. It is a lubricating organ.
It is composed of two membranes that form a virtual cavity: the pericardial cavity.

04. The Pericardium

1) The visceral bundle or epicardium, is attached to the myocardium. It extends to the coronary vessels, la grasa de los 'sillones' No entiendo esta expresión and upwards to the arterial and venal vascular pedunculi.
2) The parietal layer is fused to and inseparable from the fibrous Pericardium.
The two layers extend to the level of the line of reflection.

The fibrous Pericardium: it surrounds the serous Pericardium.
It is a thick fibrous membrane that is fused to the parietal layer of the serous membrane. The outer facial sheath of this pericardial sac is reinforced by two layers of collagenous fibres. The pericardial sac has a limited elasticity and counters an exaggerated dilation of the heart. This sac is attached to the walls by connective tissue which anchors the heart."
Anatomy and physiology books commonly say that the Pericardium is not elastic, and in itself it is not, but the crisscrossed nature of the collagenous fibres give it a certain elasticity to move and change shape depending on connective tissue retraction.

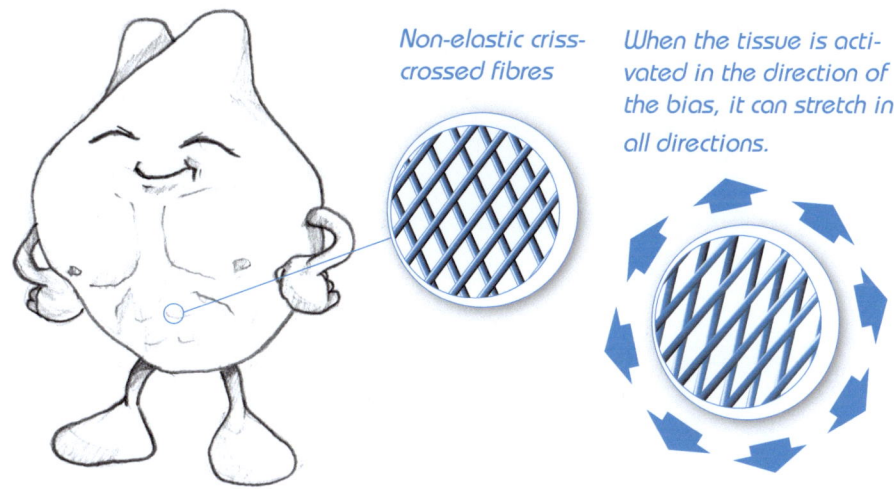

Non-elastic crisscrossed fibres

When the tissue is activated in the direction of the bias, it can stretch in all directions.

It's like a tissue that is not elastic, but it becomes so if it is stretched in the direction of the bias.

4.3 What is the purpose of the Pericardium?

The Pericardium protects and anchors the heart in its place.

The optimal functioning of the Pericardium is indispensable for LIFE, for our life, for our health.
In Chinese Medicine the Pericardium is called "The Master of the Heart".
Important Anatomy and Physiology books define the Pericardium in the following ways:
The main role of the Pericardium is to protect and anchor the heart:
- Physical protection by the lubrication of its interior
- Prevention from over dilating because of its fibrous sac
- Protection against chemicals and bacteria
- Protection against trauma
- Protection in case of hyper-pressure

To all of the above I would add, even at the risk of repetition:

The Pericardium is the emotional barrier of the heart, its guardian and its protective shield.

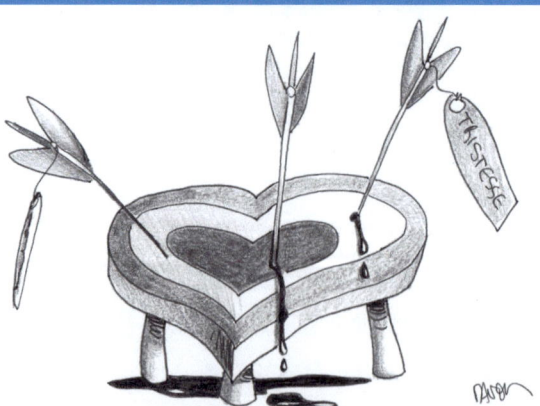

In Conclusion

Why is the Pericardium so important?
Because it contains the heart
Because of its important role in protecting the HEART
Because of its strategic location: at the centre of our body
It is between our arms and between our head and abdomen
It is between heaven and earth
Because of its direct and indirect anatomical insertions
Because of the repercussions it has on our whole health if it is dysfunctional

How does the Pericardium work?

The Pericardium is the first to receive any emotional impact. It manages it by retracting and closing up depending on the intensity of the emotion and also on the person's ability to deal with the stress. It works exactly like a cell.

This adaptive retraction to an emotional impact adds to other older, unresolved emotional shocks that are stored in the Pericardium memory. This also occurs in the cell membranes.
Consequently, the older we get and the more difficult emotional situations we have experienced, the more retracted our Pericardium becomes; it becomes hardened and closed, and it hurts.

The Pericardium stores the emotional memory of all our experiences (just like the cell membrane).

If our cells store the memory of the entire evolution of LIFE, it is evident that they can store the memories of our painful experiences!

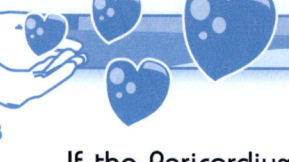

If the Pericardium is retracted, it means that we have suffered, and sometimes a lot, to the point that it closes our heart in order not to feel and suffer anymore.
At times this physiological reaction can save our life.
But if we are not able to understand this reaction, or if we are not able to resolve it and transform it, with time this accumulated retraction will cause different symptoms in order to get our attention. When that happens, it saves our life.

If we still do not want to see and understand, we get sick with different and diverse pathologies.

IT ALL COMES FROM THE SAME SOURCE

When our heart is not doing well, when we forget about our heart, closing it up and ignoring our essence as beings of LOVE, human beings, spiritual beings, it is our Pericardium that sounds the alarm to make us react so that we reconnect with the meaning of our life.

If we know how to find the meaning within our suffering, if we are able to go beyond it and to learn from each thing that happens to us, we will learn to live every circumstance of our lives as a gift, which can be more or less enjoyable, depending on our attitude. We will be able to see that the only purpose of each experience we have is to help us grow and develop as human beings.
Then, we can once again find peace in our soul (or inside our cells). Our Pericardium will be able to open and close depending on the circumstances; it will be able to adapt to these circumstances with flexibility and without complicating LIFE with the little things.

The Pericardium is the guardian of our conscience, our essence, our soul and our spirituality.

It is our Jiminy Cricket.

04. The Pericardium

4.4 Where is the Pericardium located?

In the center.

The Pericardium/heart is located in the centre plane at the mid-line of the body.

It is between our arms. Our arms and our hands work to communicate, touch, take, heal, feed, and caress, and they are directly related to our heart.

The heart suffers when we cannot hold a loved one in our arms; we talk about holding someone close to our heart.

> The heart is the first organ to form in the embryo and the first one to stop when we die.

A little anatomy

I cite again the academic sources on anatomy in order to help the reader understand the foundation of my approach, which is based on anatomical and neurophysiological observations. In the following chapters I will draw some conclusions based on my work.

ANATOMY RELATED TO THE PERICARDIUM:

In front: with the chest wall, the mediastinal pleura and lungs, which are situated between the Pericardium and the wall.

Behind: with the organs of the upper mediastinum, especially the esophagus.

Laterally: slightly separated from the mediastinal pleura by a thin soft tissue layer that contains the phrenic nerves and vessels of the upper diaphragm.

Below: it rests on the phrenic centre of the diaphragm, and it is separated from it by adipose cellular tissue.

Above: the fibrous sac separates from the parietal layer along the serous reflection line and extends over the surface of the great vessels becoming fused with the outer layer."

04. The Pericardium

HOW THE PERICARDIUM IS ATTACHED

Sternopericardial Ligaments:

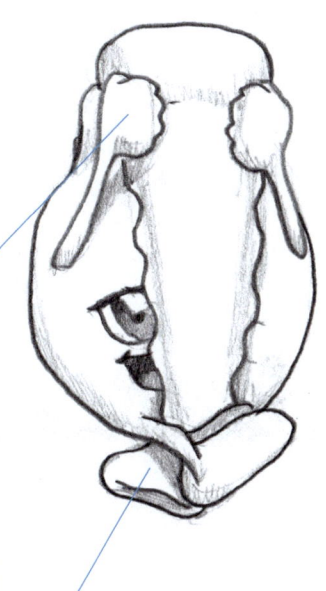

Superior: it extends from the posterior face of the manubrium of the sternum and the first two condro-sternal articulations to the antero-superior part of the Pericardium, just in front of the great vessels. It reaches down and back and is flat. It forms a triangular, vertical and frontal plate. It is a prolongation of the deep plate of the middle cervical aponeurosis.
Between the sternum and the Pericardium is the thymus.

Inferior: it extends from the inferior extremity of the sternum and the xiphoid process to the anterior wall of the pericardial sac. It lies medial and sagittal, and reaches backward. It forms a triangular and horizontal plate.

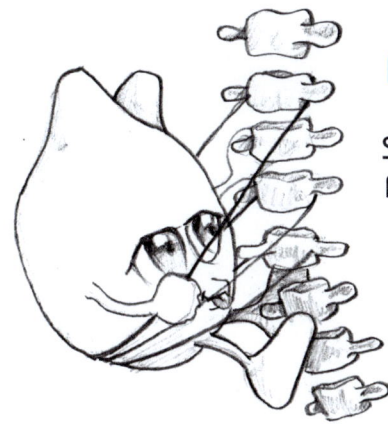

Vertebral – Pericardial ligaments:

Superior pericardial vertebral ligament from the 6th to the 7th cervical vertebrae.

Inferior pericardial vertebral ligament from the 1st to the 4th dorsal vertebrae.

(The brachial plexus is directly influenced by these ligaments.)

These fibres descend downward and forward and they end in:
The right superior in the pulmonary artery
The left superior in the carotid artery
The inferiors over the lateral face of the left auricula

Phrenic pericardial ligaments

They are extensions of the endothoracic fascia (a fibrous layer that covers the parietal surface of the pleura)

Anteriorly: it forms a V and connects the anterior base of the Pericardium with the anterior layer attached to the phrenic centre.
To the right: it fixes the Pericardium to the right of the phrenic centre.
To the left: it fixes the left posterior border of the Pericardium to the posterior aspect of the inferior vena cava.

All three attach the pericardial sac to the phrenic centre leaving a space for slipping movement: **the portal space**.

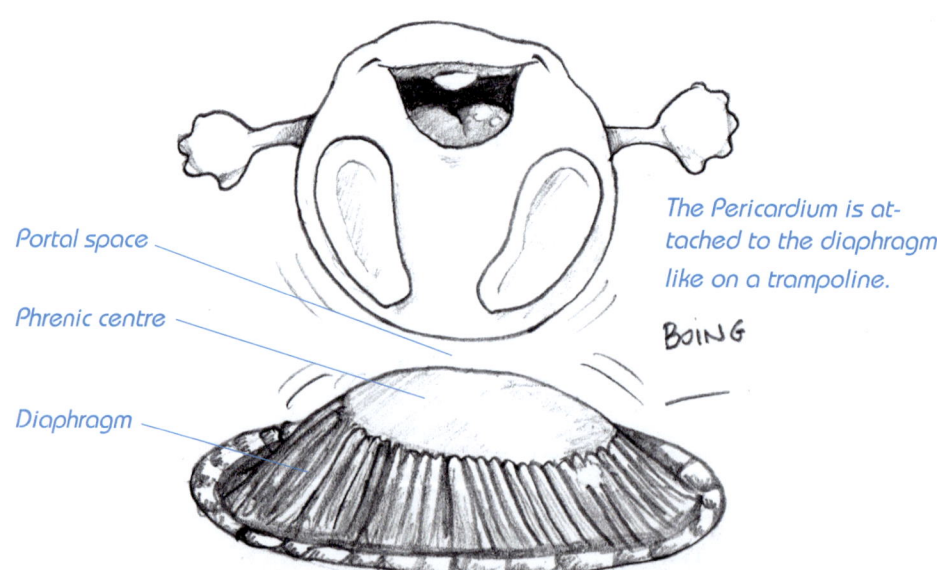

Portal space
Phrenic centre
Diaphragm

The Pericardium is attached to the diaphragm like on a trampoline.

BOING

04. The Pericardium

Thyroid pericardial ligament:

Extended between anterior surface of the Pericardium and the inferior border of the Thyroid. It envelops the brachio-cephalic venous trunk.
From above one can confuse it with the visceral sheet of the neck that inserts at the base of the cranium over the pharyngeal tubercles in the basilar area of the occiput.
It transmits all the mediastinus unbalances to the neck and to the base of the cranium.
It unites the Pericardium to the base of cranium.
It forms a posterior layer from the sac that contains the thymus that is located between the thyroid-pericardial sheet posteriorly and the superior sterno-pericardial ligament anteriorly.

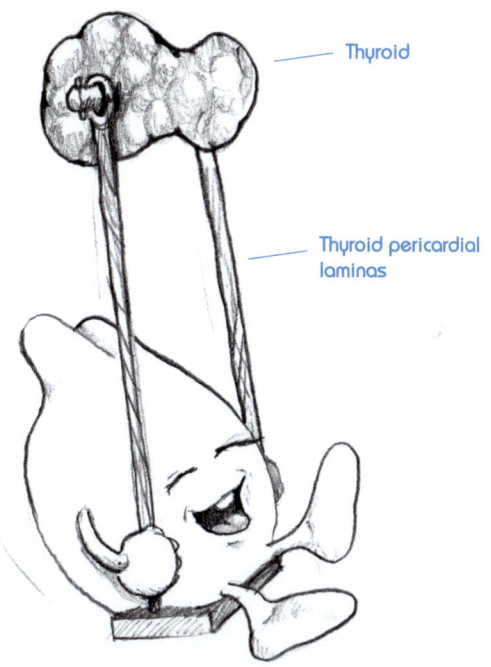

The Pericardium swings from the thyroids by the thyroid pericardial ligaments.

Visceral pericardial ligament:

They are fibrous tracts that connect the Pericardium with the esophagus, the trachea, the bronchials, and the pulmonary veins. They are not important from a fixation or attachment point of view but are very important from a functional point of view.

Anatomically, the Pericardium is the only organ that is related to the vertebral joints:

Occiput / Atlas: Through the thyroid pericardial plate that extends along the visceral sheath of the neck and inserts in the basilar area of the occiput (over the pharyngeal tubes).

Cervical Dorsal: Through the vertebral – pericardial ligaments.

Dorsal / Lumbar: Through the supports of the diaphragm.

Lumbar / Sacral: Through the aponeurosis of the pillars of the diaphragm and continuing to the iliospsoas muscle.

Anatomical Summary

Organs and other elements that are directly related with the Pericardium and are directly influenced by its functioning are:

- The mediastinal pleuras, the lungs and trachea.
- The esophagus and the opening of the stomach.
- The superior diaphragmatic vessels, the pulmonary artery and veins, the aortic arch, the left auricle, the interior vena cava, the portal vein, the brachio-cephalic venous trunk.
- The phrenic centre of the diaphragm.
- The sternum and the first two condro-sternal articulations.
- The first two ribs.
- From the Atlas to the 4th dorsal vertebrae, the brachial plexus.
- The occiput and cranial base.
- The thyroid.
- The thymus.
- The phrenic nerves that are sensitive and neurovegetative motor nerves and act on the inferior vena cava and right suprarenal capsule.

The stellate ganglion or cervicodorsal sympathetic ganglia is part of the neurovegetative nervous system, also called the autonomic nervous system.

04. The Pericardium

A little more of Anatomy

The autonomic nervous system ANS or Neuro Vegetative System: is unconscious, involuntary and independent from the Central Nervous System CNS, even though they are closely related.
It works to maintain the function of the organism's internal system – its nutrition, metabolism, adaptation and reproduction.
It keeps us in Homeostasis that means the metabolic equilibrium (balance) of a person. It has two synergic and complementary systems:
- The sympathetic system
- The parasympathetic system

A little more in depth
(if anatomy bores you, skip this part)

The superior neurovegetative centres are:

- The sub-orbital cortex and the pre-frontal cortex: regulatory centres of the psyche, consciousness and of the vegetative states.

- The Thalamus: it is a true alarm system of our organism. It receives the sensory information and it analyses it before transmitting it to the cerebral cortex, when there are stimuli that provoke fear it turns on the alarm system.

- The Hypothalamus: located below the thalamus and below the hypophysis and united to it by the pituitary trunk. It regulates our water metabolism and our sleep, it is our thermic regulator and it acts upon our awareness and over our psyche. It regulates the secretion of hormones that come from the hypophysis. It secretes antidiuretic hormones or vasopressin that controls the water in our system (organism) and also controls the oxytocin hormone which is considered to be the love hormone (see Dr. Michel's Odent work for more on this theme). It also stimulates the uterine contraction during birth and during orgasms.

- **The Hypophesis:** (or pituitary gland) is covered by the dura matter, by the tentorium cerebellum and the walls cavernous sinus. Vascularised by the ramifications of the internal carotid artery, it is the director of the orchestra of our hormonal system. It controls the thyroid, the corticosuprarrenal glands, the gonads, the basal metabolism, the sexual functions, growth, the pancreas, water balance and breast milk (feeding).

- **The Epiphysis or Pineal Gland:** (Descartes considered it to be the house of the soul and in the Hindu culture it is the location of the third eye.) It segregates melatonin and inhibits the actions of the hypothalamus and the hypophesis over the sexual glands and has an influence over the hormonal mechanisms of reproduction: the production of sperm and the menstrual cycle.

- **White matter pathways:** They are pathways of association and conduction of the cortical influx of the inter or intra-hemispheres. Its action is very important in the transmission of influx of psychic or sensorial origin to the superior neurovegetative centres. Located between them are the corpus callosum and the rhinencephalon.

- **The reticular substance:** Located in the encephalic trunk, between the nucleus of cranial nerves and the great ascending and descending pathways. It regulates the sleep-wakefulness cycle as well as concentration and learning. One needs to activate the cortex for concentration but we also need to select the information consciously; this is done by the activity of the reticular substance.

- **The neurovegetative nuclear and the cranial nerves**
Among other things, regulate the functions of cranial nerves:
- Meiosis / mydriasis
- Secretion of the salivary glands and parotid glands
- Secretion of the oral-pharyngeal mucosa
- Sensitivity of the tongue
- Lachrymal gland secretion
- Nasal mucus secretion

04. The Pericardium

I would like to make a VERY SPECIAL mention and take your attention to the star of our body; not well known but very important:

THE STELLATE GANGLION

The Stellate ganglion alone is able to overthrow our body when something goes wrong with the Pericardium.

Ansa Subclavia: Emerges from the intermediate sympathetic ganglion, it descends and wraps around the subclavian artery and continues just below to the sympathetic stellate ganglion (cervicodorsal).

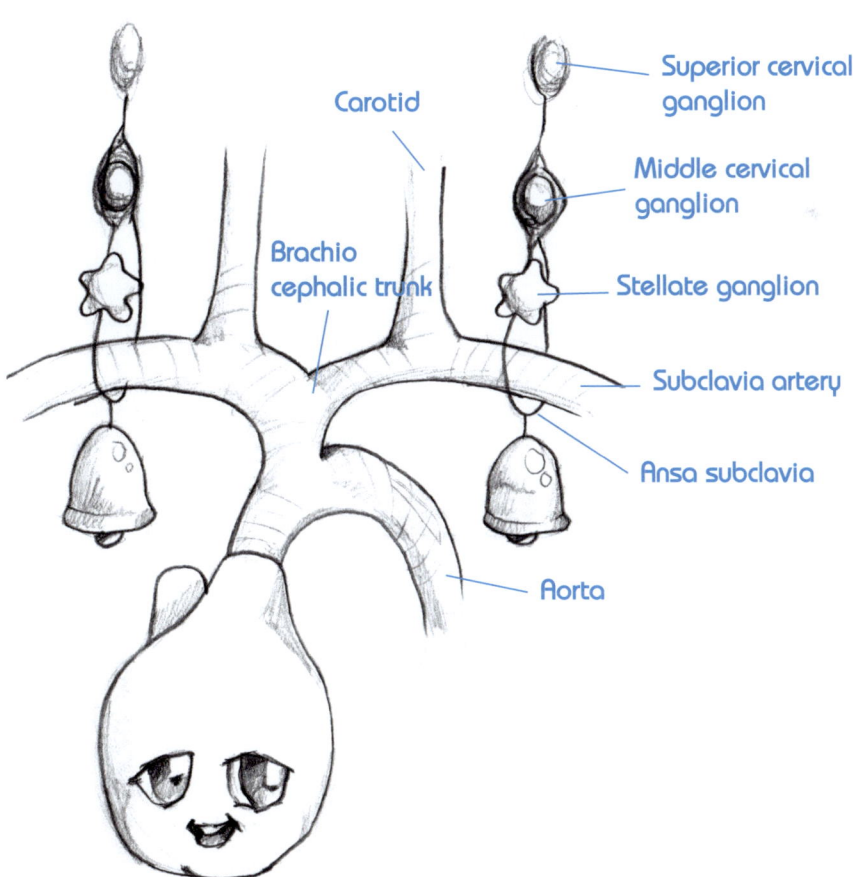

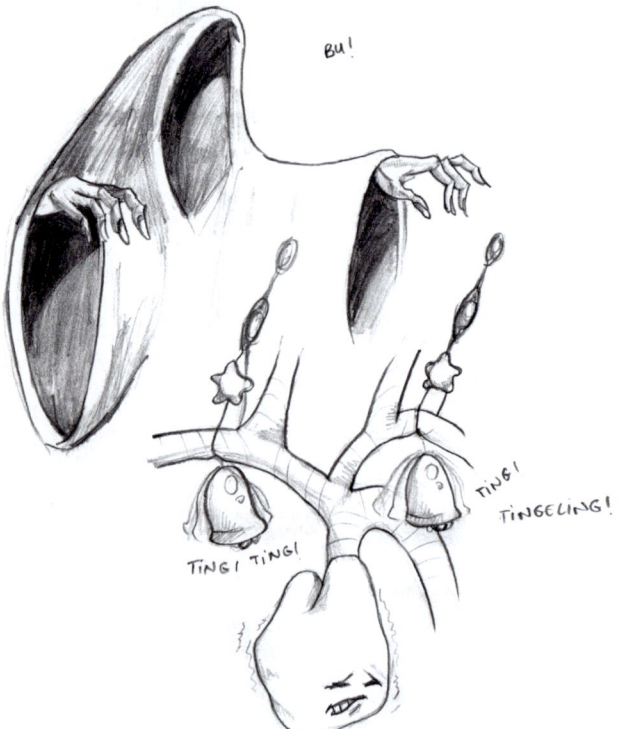

When faced with emotional stress, the Pericardium retracts and protects the heart and saves our life.

But...

When it retracts it pulls down on the bronchiocephalic trunk towards the ansa subclavia as if it were an alarm bell that wakes up all the sympathetic system starting from the stellate ganglion.

The Stellate ganglion pulls from the intermediate ganglion; this in turn pulls on the middle cervical ganglion and this one pulls on the superior cervical ganglion. The superior cervical ganglion acts on the encephalic trunk, the associated pathways, the epiphysis, the hypophysis, the hypothalamus, the thalamus, the cortex and the tonsil.

In this way it creates an alarm chain reaction that has an affect on the whole organism.

Through my observations and daily practice, I discovered that all the sympathetic fibers are interconnected and are situated strategically behind the Pericardium and below the aortic arch. Just like the ansa subclavia which are made to capture the slightest reaction of the Pericardium and be able to immediately transmit the information to the limbic system.

04. The Pericardium

Depending on the nature or the intensity of the emotional impact and the reaction at the level of the ansa subclavia, the stellate ganglion, the sympathetic system can become excited or inhibited, expressing different and diverse symptoms.

The slightest emotion provokes a retraction reaction of the Pericardium that transmits instantly to the anatomic nervous system creating an intense and a generalised reaction with a massive discharge of the sympathetic system: adrenaline.

The real pathway of our emotions starts precisely in the Pericardium, which pulls on the stellate ganglion, activating the sympathetic nervous system. Observing anatomy in this way, we can see that nature is truly wonderful.

Summing up and looking again at the scheme of Dr. David Servan Schreiber in his book The emotional cure (Ed. Kairós):

1) Fear makes the Pericardium react, 2) by retracting it pulls on the stellate ganglion, 3) it sends sympathetic information to the cardio respiratory centre of the encephalic trunk, 4) from there the stimulus goes to the thalamus and reaches the tonsil, 5) and then into the cerebral cortex.

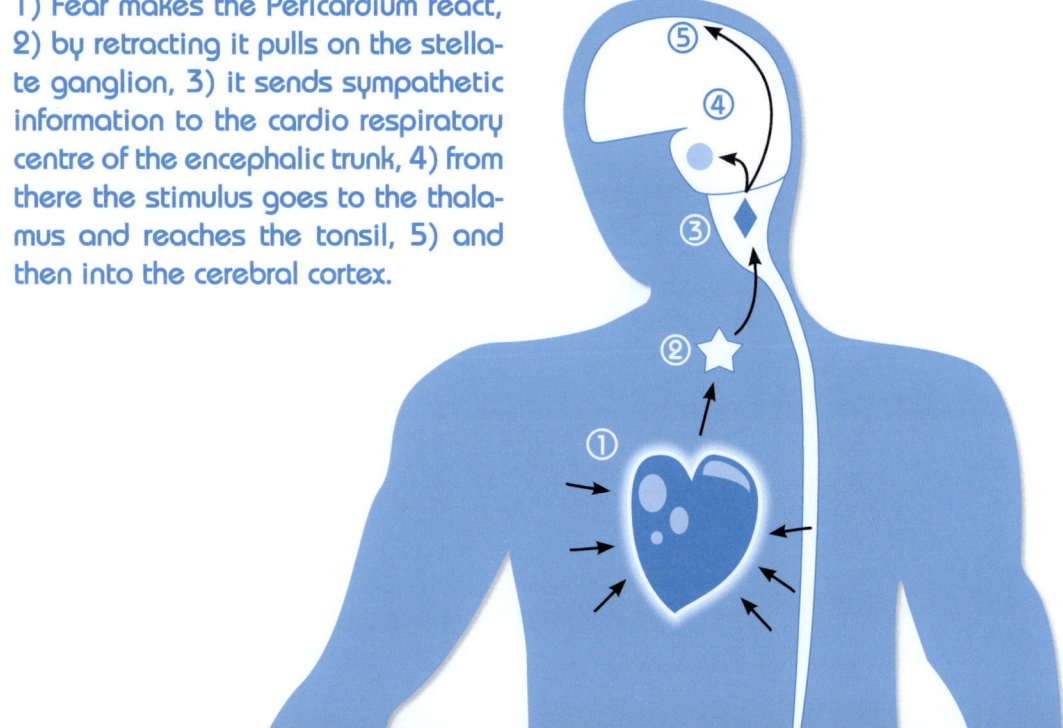

4.6 When the Pericardium is well, all goes well!
But when it does not...

Thanks to the special protection of the Pericardium the heart can be relaxed, calm and keep its vital function, even through strong emotional stress.

The Pericardium saves our life in the moment of an emotional trauma.

Due to its strategic situation, at the centre of the body, it is easy to imagine how its malfunction would disturb all the elements that compose it.

But...

When facing an emotional trauma, which can be at times even more violent and painful than a blow to the sternum:
1) The Pericardium reacts by retracting itself for protection (exactly like a cell).
2) This retraction causes a shortening in one or more of the ligaments that attach and fix the Pericardium.
3) This will have a direct repercussion on the organs, glands, vessels, nerves, membranes, muscles, bones, and other neighbouring or distant elements.

Each person reacts differently to emotional stress. Even in cases of similar situations the reactions are varied among different people. For example, faced with divorce or mourning: one person suffers a depression, the other has an heart attack, a torticollis, lumbar pain, vertigo or a knot in the stomach, someone else might get constipated, other people could have difficulty breathing or develop asthma, insomnia, some get thinner, others gain weight, others may have vision or auditory problems and still others may feel relieved and are able to finally breathe deeply, etc.

Every person is unique and when he/she is faced with the same stimulus and each one reacts in their own way, depending on their experience and the experience of their parents and ancestors... in sum, depending on their particular history.

The interesting thing is that all are affected in the same place:

In the heart / Pericardium

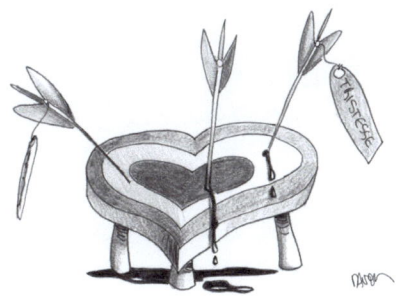

Based on the anatomy I just described to you in a summarised but practical manner (and I hope that I was clear enough), I will now describe in detail several symptoms that a Pericardium in dysfunction (one that does not work correctly) can cause.

Evidently this list is endless, and, as you will be able to see, it includes pathologies that are often called "functional", "essential" or "idiopathic", which in other words means that no physical or structural lesion can explain their existence. A dysfunction or a functional illness is when there is an organ that does not work properly, but it is not physically affected.

Statistically, it is said that 80% of all illness or pathologies are called "functional".

1/Cardiovascular disorders:

Arrhythmias, tachycardia, extrasystole, decompensated arterial tension, hypertension, cardiac murmurs

All these phenomena can be caused by a compression, strain or torsion of the Pericardium that has repercussions in its insertion at the level of the aorta.
This in turn can affect:
- the valve function, that can provoke estenosis or aortic insufficiency.
- the baroreceptors and mecanorreceptors that are located in the Aorta, on the carotid, in the subclavia artery, affecting blood pressure and the functioning of the heart.
- the cardio respiratory centre located in the encephalic trunk.
- the cardiac nerve that comes directly from the stellate ganglion.

Upper limb edema, paresthesias (the feeling of pins and needles) in the hands and upper limbs, tension differences between left and right arms

These symptoms can be caused by:
- Compression of the brachial plexus by the first rib.
- Dysfunction of the stellate ganglion which forms a sympathetic nerve bundle that envelops the subclavian artery and disturbs its motricity by vasoconstriction or vasodilation.

Intrathoratic aorta dilatation

The retraction of the phrenic-pericardial ligaments that close the diaphragm and compress the aorta do not allow the blood to flow freely, thus causing hypertension and/or intrathoracic aortic dilatation.

Aorta Dissection

When the aorta is in torsion the continuous abnormal impact by the blood pressure on its internal layer can cause an aortic dissection.

2/ Digestive disorders:

Dysphagia (difficulty in swallowing) pseudo hiatal hernia, "heaviness" at the epygastrial level, reflux, digestive difficulties, gastritis, esophagitis, caused by a compression of the Pericardium on the esophagus or on the stomach entrance.

Pericardial pain during defecation, Caused by stimulating the phrenic nerve.

The sensation of having a lump in the throat, caused by tension in the mediastinum.

Esophagitis: Caused by an irritation of the sympathetic bundle that comes out of the stellate ganglion.

3/ Respiratory disorders:

Dyspnea (difficulty taking a deep breath) sighs, sharp pains on the side with inspiration, irritative dry cough, caused by a compression of the phrenic nerve and retraction of the rib wall.

Spontaneous pneumothorax: When the Pericardium retracts, it pulls on the pleura and creates tension. If the traction is too hard, it can cause a condition known as spontaneous pheumothorax.

Asthma: Caused by inhibition of the phrenic nerve which is the nerve for inspiration.

Tracheitis: Caused by irritation of the sympathetic bundle that comes out of the stellate ganglion.

4/ Skeletal-muscular disorders:

Sternal pain: Due to a retraction of the sternopericardial ligament.

Pericardial pain with irradiation to the arm (similar to angina), due to the retraction of the superior sternopericardial ligament which closes the first two ribs and compresses the brachial plexus.

Intercostal pain: Mainly from the first to the fourth ribs, due to the tension of the vertebra-pericardial ligaments and the superior sternopericardial ligaments which close the intercostal spaces, thus compressing the intercostal nerves.

Lower cervical and upper dorsal pains: The sensation of carrying a heavy rock around the neck because of the tension in the vertebral pericardial ligaments.

Pseudo carpal tunnel syndrome, tenosynovitides of flexors, cubital tunnel syndrome: As a consequence of a compression of the C8 nerve root by the first rib.

5/ Hormonal disorders:

Hyperthyroidism, hypothyroidism, growth disorder, sexual disorders, etc.: Caused by a pull or compression of the thyroid gland through the thyroidpericardial ligament.

By an action upon the sphenobasilar symphisis, pharynx aponeurosis tract, with repercussion on the hypophysis and the epiphysis or stellate ganglion tract to the hypophysis and the thalamus, with a direct influence over the hormonal system.

Because of a retraction of the phrenic pericardial ligament that closes and compresses the diaphragm with its supports that are the suprarenal arterials.

6/ Imune System disorders:

Direct action over the thymus and spleen: The retraction of the sternopericardial ligament compresses the thymus and the spleen reducing the production of T lymphocytes.

Blockage of the rib cage and decrease in the production of blood cells in bone marrow of the ribs: The dysfunction of the phrenic nerve produces a difficulty in breathing. Little by little the patient breathes more shallowly and from the stomach. As a consequence the rib cage reduces its normal movements of respiration and the hematopoietic function of the ribs diminishes (30% of the global function).

Reduction of immunoglobin A secretion: A continuous sympathetic neurovegetative excitation provokes a reaction at the skin and mucous level decreasing the production of immunoglobin A which is part of the first line of the body's defence mechanism in the mucous of the nose, throat, bronchi, intestine and vagina, and can provoke, in turn, an immune deficiency.

7/ Lymphatic disorders:

Adenoid pathologies, lymphomas, lymphoedemas: By a compression on the Pecquet cistern due to the action of the phrenic pericardial ligaments on the diaphragm and its pillars.

By a compression of the passage of the thoracic channel through the first left rib due to a retraction of the Pericardium that pulls on the sub-clavical artery, or through a retraction of the upper right sternopericardial ligament which can produce a plugging up of the mediastinum lymph system, increasing the volume of the mediastinum ganglions.

8/ Postural disorders:

False short leg: Due to the diaphragmatic tension transmitted to the pillars with repercussion on the psoas muscle, the pelvis and the lower extremity.

Scoliosis, cifosis, lordosis: The vertebral column adapts and follows the Pericardium/Heart to protect it. Through the retractions of the ligaments it will create a scoliotic rotation to the right or to the left and a pronounced cifosis.

9/ Visual disorders:

Aniscoria, tearing, conjunctivitis, loss of acute vision: Due to an inhibition of the sympathetic nerve bundles that come from the stellate ganglion and torsion of the cranial base with repercussion at the level of the sphenord cavity.

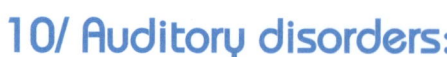

10/ Auditory disorders:

Tinnitus, functional hypoacusis, otalgia, etc.: Due to the action of the scalene muscles on the first and second ribs and the transverse apofisis from vertebras C2 to C7. The scalene muscle continues upwards toward the large muscle of the neck which inserts itself below the basilar portion of the occipital and causes a dysfunction of the cranial base and the petrous portion of the temporal bone.

Caused by the sternocleidomastoid muscle pulling the mastoid process which has a repercussion on the petrous portion of temporal bone, the petrobasilar sutures and jugular foramen through where the cranial nerves IX-X-XI, the inferior petrous sinus, the internal jugular vein and the sigmoid sinus pass.

Perception deafness, vertigo and balance problems

In the interior of the petrous portion one can find the auditory nerve (cranial nerve VIII), that is formed by the union of two nerves: the cochlear that takes care of auditory (hearing) and the vestibular nerve that is for equilibrium. In the case of incorrect functioning of the cochlear nerve a person can suffer perception deafness, if the vestibular nerve is affected a person can suffer equilibrium problems and vertigo.

11/Neurological disorders:

Vertigo: In the case of a dysfunction of the petrous portion of the temporal bone with repercussion over the vestibular nerve, forms of vertigo can manifest, called Ménier's disease with: tinnitus, deafness and falls due to instability.

Facial Neuralgia, trigeminal neuralgia, etc.: Due to petrous portion of the temporal bone dysfunction.

Epileptic type dysfunction: With or without an epileptic source. Due to a tension with torsion of the intracranial membranes that causes a partial or total compression of the cerebrum. In case of stress this dysfunction can get worse and cause convulsions.

Cervical-brachial neuralgia: Due to a compression of the brachial plexus at the level of the first rib.

Other degenerative diseases of the nervous system: Due to poor cerebral vascuralisation. From the stellate ganglion emerge two nerve bundles that envelope the vertebral and carotid arteries, responsible for cerebral vascularisation. In case of excitation or inhibition of this ganglion these nerve bundles provoke a vasoconstriction or vasodilatation of these arteries directly affecting the cerebral blood irrigation.

12/Craneal disorders:
Migraines, optic migraines, headaches
When the Pericardium retracts it pulls on its insertions in the pharyngeal apofisis, putting the sphenobasilar symphisis in extension and closing the jugular foramen. (Where the inferior petrous sinus, the internal jugular vein and the sigmoid sinus pass through.)
Bad occlusion:
Due to tension of the scalene and the sternocleidomastoid muscle, torsion is created at the cranial base, putting the temporomadibular joint in dysfunction.
Due to sphenobasilar symphisis extension which pulls down underneath the sphenoid palatine process and the two palatine bones closing the palate and the maxilar sinus.

13/Hematologie disorders:
Anemia, thrombocytopenia, alterations in the blood formula:
Due to dysfunction in the ribs and the decreasing capacity to produce red blood cells.
With each respiratory movement, especially with inspiration, the ribs move and stimulate the hematopoietic function which consists of one third of the total blood cell production. When the Pericardium and the phrenic nerve are blocked, the thoracic respiratory movements decrease and the ribs produce fewer blood cells. This can produce anemia, alteration of platelets and white blood cells along with other "inexplicable" alterations.

14/Behavioural disorders:
- sadness, depression, sorrow, anguish, negativism, anxiety
- desire to die
- aggressiveness
- feeling of having a heavy or unclear head
- panic attacks

Branches from the stellate ganglion accompany the blood vessels and cranial nerves to the limbic system and superior neurologic formations that are directly related with our emotions via the secretion of serotonin.

15/Sleep disorders:
- altered or light sleep
- insomnia
- nightmares

The traction of the Pericardium at the level of the occipital groove causes a compression of the reticular substance that is located in the encephalic trunk, which manages the sleep and wakefulness cycles.
The sphenobasilar symphisis in extension puts a tension on the intracranial membranes that insert in the pituitary and envelope the epiphysis and hypophysis. The excitation / inhibition of the epiphysis can provoke an imbalance in the melatonin secretion and cause consequences in sleep regulation.

4.7 Perspectives from other Medical Traditions
On the Pericardium

Chinese Medicine

After understanding the vital importance of the Pericardium for the human organism, I began making an endless series of realisations and confirmations that have surprised me day after day and encouraged me to continue delving into this vision of health.
I became interested in how other medicines viewed the Pericardium. Here is what I found:

The Pericardium is the "Master Heart"

I will quote now some very interesting words from the book The Fundamental Principles of Chinese Medicine by MACIOCIA,

"The Functions of the Master Heart":
The Master Heart (meridian of the Pericardium) is intimately related to the heart. Traditionally, the function of the Master of the heart has been considered to be that of external protection of the heart against external pathogenic attacks. In chapter 71 of The Spiritual Axis it says that the heart is the emperor that governs the five yin and the six yang viscera; it houses the Spirit and it is so hard that no pathogen factor can install itself there. If the heart is attacked by a pathogen factor the spirit will suffer and it may even result in death.

"The Heart is the Emperor" and "the Master of the Heart is the Ambassador:
It governs joy and happiness"

"According to the Visceral Theory the functions of the Master of the Heart are almost the same as the Heart:

- It Governs the blood
a) It is at the heart level that the transformation of the Qi (or Chi) elements from food into the blood takes place.
b) The heart is responsible for making the blood circulate.

- It Houses the Spirit
According to Chinese medicine both mental activity and consciousness "live" in the heart, which means that the heart has repercussions on mental activities as well as on the emotional states of the individual. Five functions are particularly affected by the state of the heart:

- Mental activities
- Emotions
- The conscience
- Memory
- Thought
- Sleep

From the perspective of the meridians, the Master of the Heart meridian is very different from that of the heart. Its sphere of influence is very specific and is located mostly in the centre of the thorax."

"Like the heart, the Master of the Heart also has an influence on the relationships that one has with others, and its meridian points are frequently used when treating emotional problems related to relationship difficulties". (p.104 y 151)

It is through the Meridians that Chinese medicine elaborates the connections of the Pericardium at the anatomical level and their repercussions at the physiological level. With this view, the two medicine traditions join together and complement each other.

Ayurvedic Medicine

I have not found citations in Ayurvedic medicine that mention the Pericardium specifically. But a few years ago I read a book written by Dr. Deepak Chopra *"Vivre la Sante"* (Montreal, Stanke, 1988), when I had not yet begun my research on the Pericardium.

Chopra describes different syndromes in this very interesting book, but what caught my attention in particular was the Burn Out Syndrome.

Burn Out according to Dr. Deepak Chopra:

"Fatigue, headaches, insomnia, lumbar pain, digestive problems, respiratory difficulties, persistent flues, weight gain or loss. They are able to survive by rationalizing their behaviour, being absorbed in activities and thoughts of obsessive character: irritable, tense, cynical and picky."

What a simple and complete way to describe a Pericardium in dysfunction!

Energy Medicine

Energetic medicine works with the body through the chakras. The heart chakra is called ANAHATA, and it is the centre of LOVE energy, of the higher emotions. It is the centre of the essential being. This centre is related to the archetype of human compassion. This chakra develops after change in conscience when one transcends his or her being to connect with someone else.

When the emotional energy is properly channelled it turns into pure LOVE and devotion (Bhakti).

It is at the ANAHATA level that acceptance and unconditional love towards someone is born; pure love without any expectations. This state shows us our way of relating to the world.

I quote from the book "Anatomy of the Spirit" by Carol Myss.
"**The fourth Chakra: The Power of the Emotions**
The fourth Chakra is the central powerhouse of the human energy system. It intermediates between the body and spirit and determines their health and strength. Fourth chakra energy is affectionate by nature and nourishes our development in this plane. This chakra embodies the spiritual lesson that teaches us how to act out of love and compassion and recognise that the most powerful energy we have is love.
Location: centre of the chest.
Energy connection between the energy body and the physical body: this chakra vibrates the tuning fork of our emotions that determines the quality of our lives far more than our mental perceptions. As children, we react to our circumstances with a wide range of emotions: love, compassion, confidence, hope, despair, hate, envy and fear. As adults, we are challenged to generate within ourselves an emotional climate and steadiness from which to act consciously and with compassion.
Symbolic and perceptual connection: More than any other chakra, the fourth chakra represents our capacity to "let go and let God". With its energy we accept our personal emotional challenges as extensions of a Divine plan, which has as its intent our conscious evolution. By releasing our emotional pain, by letting go of our need to know why things happen as they have, we reach a state of tranquillity. In order to achieve that inner peace, however, we have to embrace the healing energy of forgiveness and release our lesser need for human, self-determined justice.
Sefirot and the sacraments connection: The fourth chakra corresponds to the Sefirot of Tif'eret, symbolic of the beauty and compassion within God. This energy represents the heart of the Divine – an endless pouring forth of the nurturing life force. The sacrament of marriage is congruent to the energy of the fourth chakra. As an archetype, marriage represents first and foremost a bond with oneself, the internal union of self and soul.
The challenge inherent in the fourth chakra is similar to that of the third but is more spiritually sophisticated. While the third chakra focus is on our feeling about ourselves in relation to our physical world, the fourth chakra focuses on our feelings about our internal world – our

emotional response to our own thoughts, ideas, attitudes and inspirations, as well as the attention we give to our emotional needs. This level of commitment is the essential factor in forming healthy relationships with others.

Primary fears: Fears of loneliness, commitment and "following one's heart"; fear of inability to protect oneself emotionally; fear of emotional weakness and betrayal. Loss of fourth chakra energy can give rise to jealousy, bitterness, anger, hatred, and an inability to forgive others as well as to forgive oneself.

Primary strengths: Love, forgiveness, compassion, dedication, inspiration, hope, trust, and the ability to heal oneself and others.

Sacred truth: The fourth chakra is the power centre of the human energy system because Love Is Divine Power. While intelligence or "mental energy" is generally considered superior to emotional energy, actually emotional energy is the true motivator of the human body and spirit. Love in its purest form – unconditional love – is the substance of the Divine, with its endless capacity to forgive and respond to our prayers. Our own hearts are designed to express beauty, compassion, forgiveness and love. It is against our spiritual nature to act otherwise.

We are not fluent in love, but we spend our life learning about it. Its energy is pure power. We are as attracted to love as we are intimidated by it. We are motivated by love, controlled by it, inspired by it, healed by it, and destroyed by it. Love is the fuel of our physical and spiritual bodies. Each of life's challenges is a lesson in some aspect of love. How we respond to these challenges is recorded within our cell tissue: we live within the biological consequences of biographical choices."

This vision explains and completes our affirmation about the wholeness of the human being as a spiritual and energetic being whose primary fuel for its optimal development and evolution is love.

4.8 A bit of history on the Pericardium

Claude Galien (131-201 BC): He discovered and named the Pericardium for the first time. The name comes from Greek language "peri" meaning around and "kardia" meaning heart: around the heart.

A few centuries later AVENZOAR (1113-1162): An Arab doctor of Cordoba, Spain described Pericarditis in his work "Altheisir".

The Italian doctor Giorgio BAGUM (1668-1707), professor of anatomy in Rome, in his book Praxis Medica (1696) describes the calcifications of the Pericardium (concretio cardis) "as if the heart was covered by a core layer of cement."

In 1673, the French anatomist of Montpellier, Raymond VIEUSSENS (1641-1716), described the adhesions of the Pericardium and observed the limitations that they provoked in the activities of the heart. It was he who described the famous Vieussens' ansa (called today subclavian loop).

Jean-Baptiste SENAC (1693-1770), a French clinician of Versailles, wrote the first great work on anatomy, physiology and the pathologies of the heart, The Treaty of the structure of the heart, its action and diseases, written in two volumes. In the second volume he talks about the Pericardium where he writes that in case of a disease, adhesions can be formed and they will have repercussions on the heart's mechanics.

Giovanni Battista MORGAGNI (1682-1771) Italian doctor who was the most important anatomist pathologist of that time. In his work of

04. The Pericardium

five volumes On the sites and causes of disease, he tried to establish a relationship between anatomy, pathology and clinical medicine studying 700 cases and their autopsies.

He established the relationship between dysphagia and fibrous pericarditis. He also described the pericardial stroke, adhesions and calcifications.

1818 -1886: The first person to describe the treatment of obstructive chronic pericarditis was an English man named Norman CHEEVERS. In "Observation on diseases that affect the opening and valves of the aorta" (1842), he talks about the compressive effects pericardial adhesions have on the Pericardium and their systolic and diastolic reductions. He observed that chronic pericarditis adhesions often provoked an intense and recurrent ascites.

W.William STOKES (1804 -1878) of London, in his book The diseases of the heart and the aorta, he cites that the friction that one can hear in a pericarditis could be amplified if one increased lightly the pressure with the stethoscope and it could even disappear with a greater pressure. The act of rubbing could also change the intensity depending on the position of the patient and would increase when in a sitting position. He also observed that sometimes the pericarditis precedes the affects of rheumatic fever in the articulations.

Joseph SKODA (1805-1881) of Vienna perfected the "Skoda's Resonance" in order to diagnose the pericardial stroke, which is also used to clinically demonstrate constrictive pericarditis and the phenomenon that he named "diastolic heart beat". When the heartbeat has an absence of systolic impulse from the top, a systolic pericardia retraction, and a sudden diastolic drainage from the cervical veins – this constitutes a pathognomonic sign of constrictive pericarditis.

Pierre Carl Edouard POTAIN (1825 -1901), French, is known for the description of the protodiastolic sound that warns of a constrictive pericarditis.

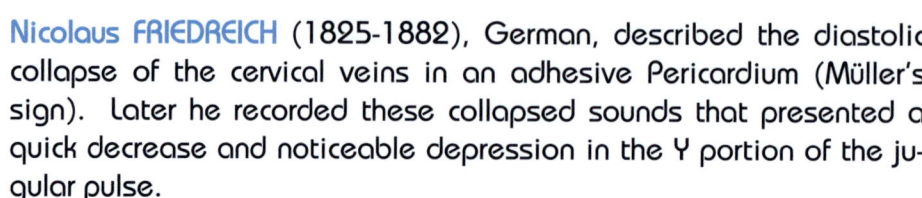

Nicolaus FRIEDREICH (1825-1882), German, described the diastolic collapse of the cervical veins in an adhesive Pericardium (Müller's sign). Later he recorded these collapsed sounds that presented a quick decrease and noticeable depression in the Y portion of the jugular pulse.

Adolf KUSSMAUL (1822-1902), German, described the "paradoxic pulse" in adhesive pericarditis (mediastino pericarditis). The Kussmaul signal is known for an increase in venous pressure during inspiration that swells the veins of the throat.

Friedel PICK (1867-1926) of Prague described the syndrome known as "Pick Disease" a pseudo cirrhosis of the liver associated with a chronic adhesive pericarditis with mediastinum affection.

Nils R.FINSEN (1860-1904), he himself was affected by constrictive pericarditis and was not treated surgically. The first symptoms appeared at age 23 with a hepatomegaly, then a systolic retraction at the apex of the heart, later a "galloping" rhythm.
At the age of 33 an auricular fibrillation appeared. He died at the age of 44 after several pericardial strokes and a number of paracentesis.

Ludolf BRAUER (1865-1951), German, who in the cases of mediastino pericarditis recommended an ostectomy of the ribs and the costal cartilages where the adhesions where found.

Paul HALLOPEAU (1876-1924), a French surgeon that preformed the first partial pericardectomy to alleviate a constrictive pericarditis. Two years later two German surgeons Franz von VOLHARD (1872-1950) and Victor SCHMIEDEN (1874-1945) performed the first total pericardectomy to improve a constrictive pericarditis.

Willem EINTHOVEN (1860-1927) from Holland, received the Nobel Prize in physiology in 1924 for developing the science of the electrocardiogram.

04. The Pericardium

Charles C. THOMAS edited The Pericardium and its Disorders, Charles C. THOMAS Publisher, Springfield, Illinois USA 1971. Spanish Edition, 1973, by Publisher TORAY of Félix M. CORTES.

In the above portion of the history of the Pericardium, I have only mentioned the authors that touched on and described in detail the condition of constrictive pericarditis. The other pericardial conditions are, in my opinion, a consequence of this initially mentioned condition. What surprises me about this history is that all of the people have described, enumerated, and confirmed the symptoms, however...

Nobody gave priority to, or questioned why the Pericardium closes up in such a way.

The only question they asked themselves was:

How am I going to threat the Pericardium?
Making a hole in it, puncturing it, aspirating it, injecting it, cutting it or simply removing it, why not?

When we understand how the Pericardium reacts and closes in the face of painful events in our lives, we can help the Pericardium to free itself so that it will function well and that we can find happiness and health. We are going to do it with the necessary love and tenderness to give it trust and alleviate its wounds so that it can let go and open up again without fear.

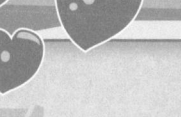

How to feel the Pericardium

If you recognise yourself in one or more of the symptoms described earlier, if you feel your heart closed, if you have been examined and told that all is normal but you still feel there is something wrong, than you can try to free your Pericardium little by little and see if that makes you feel better.

Before freeing it, it is necessary to connect with it; to feel it first in order to familiarise yourself with its presence.

For that I recommend that you perform the exercise of centring yourself from chapter one. Doing it two or three times a day is ideal not only for your Pericardium but to become centred, to re-encounter yourself and to entering contact with LIFE, with your essence and with your soul.

Exercises to feel centred and to feel LIFE:
You can do it in the morning or at any time of the day that you are calm and in silence. Sit comfortably in a calm and quiet place. Turn off the phone. Take your time; you are going to re-learn to let go like you did when you were a child.

1. Sit comfortably so that your feet are in good contact with the earth or the floor. Place the palm of your hands lightly, softly and without tension over your thighs.

2. Look for a comfortable position for your pelvis, a good cushion for your buttocks, check that your back is straight, shoulders, neck, head relaxed and loose arms.

3. When you are sitting comfortably, close your eyes and breath deeply and calmly.

04. The Pericardium

4. Let your ideas and thoughts pass by as if they were a movie that does not have anything to do with you, get them go by effortlessly, without a struggle.

5. Take your attention to your heels and their contact with the earth.

6. Visualise that there are roots coming out of your heels and your coccyx that reach down deeply into the centre of earth.

7. Visualise and feel this energy at the centre of the earth and let this energy go up through your roots, passing through your heels, up through your ankles, your legs, your pelvis.

8. Feel how this energy grows in your pelvis, moving upward into your diaphragm, over flowing into your heart and Pericardium, into your chest and your shoulders.

9. Let this energy go down your arms filling your hands and your fingers, sense how they fill up with LIFE, with vibration.

10. Let this energy go up from your heart and Pericardium to your neck, feel how it pushes your head towards the sky and how it becomes less heavy, and filled with light and life.

11. Let this energy go out like a stream of light from the centre of your cranium, up towards the sky, to infinite space.

12. SAVOUR these moments feeling yourself BETWEEN HEAVEN AND EARTH, so small like a single cell and so big as you are.

13. WITHOUT ANY STRUGGLE, feel LIFE pass through your body from the EARTH TO THE SKY and from the SKY TO EARTH. Savour it even more, there is nothing for you to do, only feel.

14. Now take your attention to the level of your Pericardium.

15. Feel the energy that comes from earth, how it passes through your heels, your legs, your pelvis, your diaphragm and feel it reach your Pericardium.

16. Let your Pericardium fill up with life, let it swell up, let it vibrate.

17. Feel the LIFE that comes from the heavens, that passes down through the top of your head and descends through you neck until it reaches the Pericardium, let the energy that comes from earth mix with the one from above. Let them dance in your chest, feel their heat and movement.

18. Enjoy, enjoy.

Now you are ready to feel.

1. Place your right hand in the middle of your chest and your left hand over your right hand.

2. Both hands are crossed and in the middle of your chest, touching lightly, floating over the Pericardium.

3. Take your attention to your Pericardium thinking only "Pericardium".

4. You can say to your Pericardium, "Pericardium show me your movement", then continue and ask "How do you feel?"

5. Your hands are floating over it, like a cork floating on water, flexible and light, but touching it enough to be able to follow the wide range of its movement and then speak the emotion you feel that your Pericardium answers to you.

6. Dance with your Pericardium to its fullest amplitude, without fear, without wavering.

7. When there is a release, you will feel a sigh come out, a deep breath... And above all,

8. Tell it, "I have treated you badly because of my lack of understanding, I got separated from who I am".

Do this exercise as many times as you feel necessary, it can only do you good. Above all do it in moments of stress, and when you feel that a situation, a word, a look, a piece of news, an image, etc., has touched you and closed your heart.

LET GO,
without struggle and with trust.

THERE IS NOTHING YOU HAVE TO DO,
just follow the movement and let it take you with it.

In case of emergency

Do the following if you have a pain in your chest and fear it could be a cardiac arrest: while you wait for the doctor or the ambulance, breath calmly and deeply; place your hands over your heart and liberate it by calming it. You can even talk to it and tell it the reason of your stress. Give thanks for the experience of life together and breathe deeply.

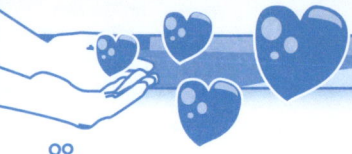

Conclusion

When the doctor gives us a serious diagnosis about our health, we have the tendency to think:
- Why did it happen to me and not to my neighbour?
- I have lived a "healthy" life, I eat correctly, I am a good person, etc.

It is our essence that gets sick, when we loose our focus, our centre... Or when we hurt our heart, when we ignore it, forget it, deny it and we hide in pure reason.

> When our soul suffers,
> **our heart / our body gets sick.**

When I distance myself from my soul, from my path of life, from my mission in this earth:

- I do not feel good
- I am unfocused
- I feel unbalanced
- I feel out of sorts
- My soul hurts
- I am sick

Illness is when my soul is closed, trapped, made smaller, blocked at the inner part of my cells and organs; when its divine and limitless potential is curtailed.

05. Conclusion

> **The Pericardium is the link between the soul, the heart and the body.**

1/ I am an unlimited spiritual being. Spiritual (which means God) is to say that I am a divine spirit.
I am made flesh to live a physical experience through my body. My mission in life will allow me to be a realised and divine person.

2/ When I forget WHO I AM I get scared.
Fear perturbs my emotional body that is in direct relation with my neuro-hormonal system.
I begin to segregate hormones of fear like adrenaline.

3/ Under the effect of adrenaline, my metabolic system becomes unbalanced and:
I feel tired, disturbed, altered, sad, etc.
As a consequence my visceral system is affected.

4/ My bad metabolic function alters and disturbs my viscera and my vital organs.
I have bad digestion, cardiovascular and immune disorders.

5/ This Visceral dysfunction causes a maladjustment at the muscular skeletal system (muscles, bones and joints).
The muscular skeletal system serves to protect and hold the vital organs, that is to say, it is at their service.
Joint pain appears, or neuralgias and tendonitis, etc. It is the muscles, tendons and joints that are the last ones in the chain!

And they are the ones we worry the most!

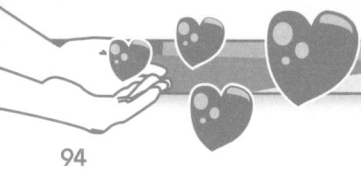

Therefore...

THE PERICARDIUM is the main door to our emotions, and evidently, to our sense organs.

If I can't see the images that cause me harm, I close my eyes or imagine a disease that stops me from seeing them.

If I don't want to hear words that hurt me, I close my ears or I create a disease that prevents me from hearing.

If I do not want to smell the odours that bother me I close my nose.

If I can't "feel" someone, than I create an illness that will prevent myself from feeling.

If I do not want to be touched, I protect myself, I get sick, I isolate myself or generate an illness so that nobody has the desire to touch me.
When my heart has been hurt due to lack of love, or abandonment, or a separation, or loss, then my Pericardium protects it by closing up and hardening like a shield so that these emotions cannot reach in. This way I won't suffer anymore.

But when I close up to EMOTIONS and to feelings I separate myself from my essence. And instead of living and vibrating, I begin to simply survive.

*I become like a robot,
without pain and without glory.*

05. Conclusion

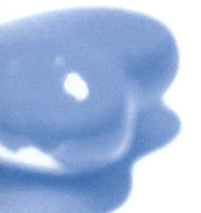

But when our Pericardium / heart is free, light, open and flexible…
We naturally feel inclined to:

Solidarity	Respect
Friendship	Happiness
Compassion	And in Conclusion…

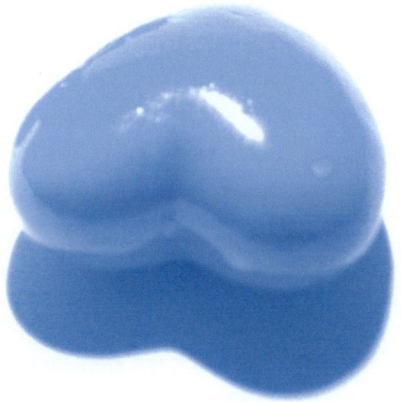

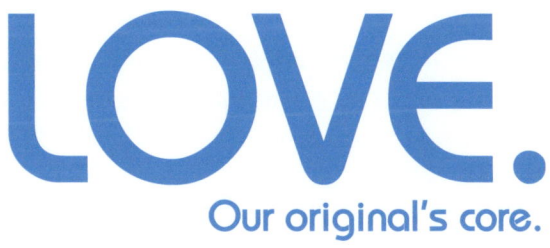

LOVE.
Our original's core.

The last centuries have been distinguished by a great development of science, technology and industry; it is the era of the brain: of reason, logic, theory, philosophy, etc. I feel that today the era of the heart is beginning: the era of emotions, of LOVE, of sharing, of respect for the human being – for ourselves as human beings and for the rest of the living beings – and for LIFE in all its manifestations.

It is about time that the heart finds its place, not only as a vital organ by excellence because of it function as a cardiac pump, but as an essential element for our balance and health.

It a time for re-encountering our heart that houses and governs our emotions, that works as a link between the different elements and systems in our body, and energetically links us to all other living beings and to the universe.

In order to help and participate in this universal movement of LOVE, we have created:

"FREE THE PERICARDIUM PEOPLE'S UNION"

A touch of humour between therapists from different countries around the world, liberators of the Pericardium and of LIFE in general.

UNION: because it unites and grows in all directions there where LIFE takes it:
PEOPLE'S: because it is reachable by all, due to its simplicity and depth. And obviously open to everyone that wants to join us on this wonderful path that consists of the liberation to HAPPINESS.

We are NOT related to any political, cultural, social or philosophical group.

We only help to free the Pericardium, so that everyone can connect to their essence and be able to find their own path in life.

05. Conclusion

THERAPIST etymologically means God's server, which means server of life or server of the soul, or whatever you want to call it.

Here is the Mission of the "Free the Pericardium People's Union":

Freeing LIFE, is freeing happiness. It means liberating the vital energy of humanity, of our human essence.

Freeing LIFE is liberating the light that helps us to see clearly so we do not get lost or distanced from our path of life.

Freeing LIFE is liberating this subtle vibrating that lets us fully enjoy our actions and our senses.

Liberating LIFE is also liberating our omnipresent intellect, the one that makes us see life with a logical, square, dogmatic point of view, without fantasy.

Freeing LIFE is liberating our heart from all our social, political, religious, intellectual barriers that we carry from childhood and that stop us from accessing our ancestral and innate wisdom that goes beyond cultural or intellectual knowledge.

Long live LIFE!!
Long live the FREE PERICARDIUM!!

Bibliography

FELIX M. CORTES
Enfermedades del Pericardio
Ed. TORAY

ISSARTEL L. et M.
L'Ostéopathie exactement
Ed. Robert Laffont, 1983

TRICOT P.
L'Ostéopathie, une thérapie à découvrir
Ed. Chiron, 1988

TRICOT P.
Ostépathie, Libére La Vida
Ed. Chiron, 1992

ANDREW TAYLOR STILL
Autobiographie
Académie d'Ostéeopathie de France, 1998

ROULIER G.
L'Ostéopathie, deux mains pour vous guérir.
Ed. Dangles, 1987

MASARU EMOTO
Los Mensajes del Agua
Ed. La Liebre de Marzo

NETTER F.
Atlas d'Anatomie humaine
Ed. Novartis, 1989

ROUVIERE H. et DELMAS A.
Anatomie humaine
Ed. Masson, 1991

DELMAS A.
Voies et centres nerveux
Ed. Masson, 1991

SILBERNAGL et DESPOPOULOS
Atlas de poche de Physiologie
Flammarion, 1979

NADER T.
La physiologie humaine l'expression du Véda

BRICOT B.
La reprogrammation posturale globale

PICANIOL G.
Les manipulations vertebrales

CORMAN L.
Visages et caractères
Ed. Puf, 1989

LOWEN A.
El amor, el sexo y la salud del corazón
Ed. Herder, 1997

G.DAVID et P.HAEGEL
Embryologie
Ed, MASSON

Ghislaine SAINT-PIERRE LANCTÔT
La mafia médicale

Ghislaine LANCTÔT
Que diable suis-je venue faire sur cette terre ?

Dr. Bernardo FERRANDO
Flores del mburucuyá de la sierra

CAROL MYSS
Anatomie de l'esprit
Livre de Poche.

CHOPRA D.
Vivre sa santé
Ed.Stanké

David SERVAN SCHREIBER
Guerir
Robert Laffont

LIEVEGOD B.
Las etapas evolutivas del niño
Ed. Rudolf Steiner, 1999

CHOPRA D.
La santé parfaite

CHOPRA D.
Le corps quantique
Ed. Altess, 1990

SINOUÉ G.
Le livre des sagesses d'Orient
Ed. 1, 2000

BEINFIELD H. y KORNGOLD E.
Entre cielo y tierra
Ed. Lievre de marzo, 1991

MACIOCIA G.
Les principes fondamentaux de la médecine chinoise
Ed. Satas, 1992

Index

Introduction	06
Chapter 1. Life	**16**
1.1. What is life?	18
1.2. Water, the source of LIFE	24
1.3. The movement of LIFE	26
1.4. Can one "feel" LIFE?	29
1.5. How can one "feel" LIFE?	30
Chapter 2. The Cell	**34**
2.1. A little biology	36
2.2. Fundamental biological laws	37
Chapter 3. Fear	**42**
Chapter 4. The Pericardium	**48**
4.1. Why the Pericardium?	50
4.2. What is the Pericardium?	54
4.3. What is the purpose of the Pericardium?	56
4.4. Where is the Pericardium located?	59
4.5. A little anatomy	60
4.6. When the Pericardium is well, all goes well!	70
4.7. Perspectives from other Medical Traditions	79
4.8. A bit of history on the Pericardium	84
4.9. How to feel the Pericardium	88
Conclusion	92

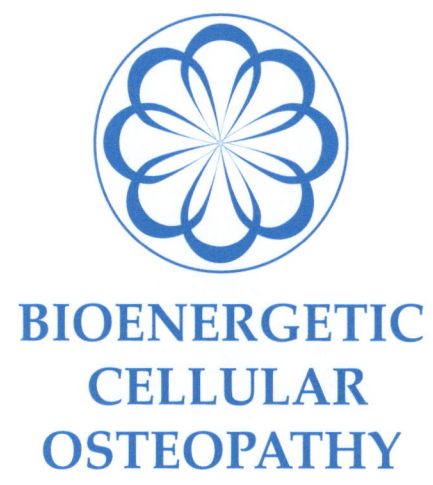

BIOENERGETIC CELLULAR OSTEOPATHY

montserratgascon@yahoo.es
www.vivalavida.org

Long live the free Pericardium !

All rights reserved

© 2011 Montserrat Gascón Segundo
c/ Llevant 74 - 6º 2º, 08402 Granollers, Barcelona
0034 93 861 36 00
montserratgascon@yahoo.es

www.vivalavida.org

Created by
Montserrat Gascón Segundo and Oriol Martinez Gascón

Third edition : January 2012

ISBN-13 : 978-2-8106-2243-6

Registration of copyright : January 2012

Production and editor

Editions : Books on Demand GmbH,
12/14 Rond-Point des Champs-Elysées, 75008 Paris, France
Imprimé par Books on DemandeGmbH, Norderstedt, Allemagne

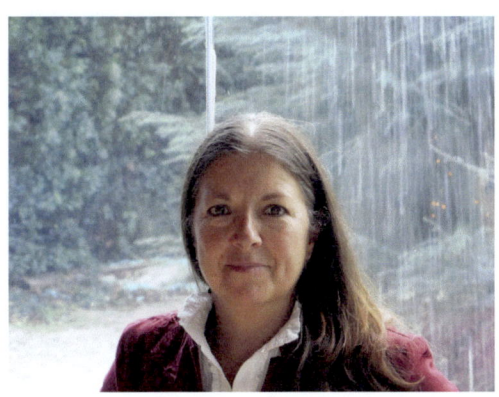

Montserrat GASCON
Born in 1953 in Granollers Barcelona Spain.

Studies : Nursing school, Medicine faculty, Morpho-psychology Professor by the École française de M.P. du Dr. Louis Corman in Paris, Osteopathy in Aix en Provence, Neurology with Dr. Nelson Annunciato,...

**I AM pure energy,
Experiencing LIFE through my body.**

Authoress of the following books :
« Long life Free Pericardium »
« Le Secret du cœur »
Fruits of my personnal, scientific and professionnal experiences.

Creator of the Bioenergetic Cellular Ostheopathy.